Sexual Predators

Serial Killers in the Age of Neuroscience

Don Jacobs

✦

Weatherford College

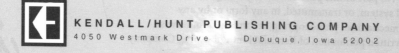

KENDALL/HUNT PUBLISHING COMPANY
4050 Westmark Drive   Dubuque, Iowa 52002

Preface

◾ The Living Nightmare of Netherworld

In North America, a percentage of family milieus are so dysfunctional that a kind of **netherworld**, or counter-culture of antisocial parenting, has developed over the past ten years or so, producing children who become violent human predators, or what society calls serial killers. Camouflaged by societal persona, *sexual predators* hide behind a reptilian brain bent upon *rapacious behavior*—preying upon others for sexual thrill. The end result, of course, is that no safe neighborhoods exist. Where can children run and play with innocent abandonment? Without parental vigil, no such place exists.

Roaming freely in society, killing a string of strangers sequentially, pedophiles, rapists, and killers have made parents uptight and almost panicky. For good reason: they target children and young women.

Antisocial parenting aside, netherworld has created a class of desensitized citizens. An increasing number of individuals (many of them parents) in the age group most populated by serial killers (25 to 39 years of age), put their heads in the sand, choosing to ignore the reality of "a brave new world" brought about by netherworld. They plunge into escapism and the trivialities offered by pop culture USA. In the meantime, their minds decay with the sweet promise of aestheticism courtesy of empty caloric intake and reality TV. Yet, parents who nurture their children do exist. A quick glance at newspaper headlines on occasion suggests their numbers might be diminishing. Yet, loving, nurturing parents make all the difference in the world to their children and to everyone else outside of netherworld.

The truth is, potential terrorism is around us everyday in shopping malls, parks, along lazy country roads, and amid thriving neighborhoods in broad daylight on busy streets. Sexual predators "hide" in the open, just outside the "frame" of our perception, waiting and watching to see if we are attentive to our beautiful children. They stalk children in department stores waiting to see if adult chaperons become inattentive, even for a few seconds. They watch checkout lines for a quick steal and rapid exit though sliding doors to an accomplice waiting at curbside with the motor running.

Species *Homo pseudo-sapien* is a reptile hiding behind a human face. When they steal children, the chance of finding them alive is the same for the serial killer's "recovery" upon capture, which is zero.

Serial killers exist in the surreal glare of a living nightmare brought about by netherworld—horrific antisocial parenting producing irreversible neurological brain damage, deviant cognitive mapping, and poly-addiction. Forensic evidence gathered at crime scenes, victimology (choice of victim), and the nature of the crime itself paint a Goya-like portrait of a *sexual deviant* who is much more than an antisocial, or a *psychopathic personality*. He is a sexual psychopath. He kills, and he will never stop.

Sexual predators kill sequentially as though guided by an ever-conscious REM clock that's ticking. In sleep, REM occurs sequentially throughout the night producing vivid fantasy (dreams) and sexual arousal. The conscious, waking hours of sexual predators eerily correspond to the sleeper's cycles of REM (vivid dreams) and NREM ("thought-like" quality of dreams). During waking "REM," the killer is sexually active, capturing and restraining his victim, preparing her for sexual experimentation and death. Soon, he will kill her. During waking "NREM"—marked by a "cooling off" period—he begins the search for another victim. He knows "REM"—the realization of his fantasy—

is coming soon; he can barely contain his sexual energy as the day moves him closer . . . closer to the complete domination of another person.

Netherworld is part of the real world. We can no longer ignore it. We must address what makes some families so dysfunctional. In the meantime, we must become more vigilant if we want out children to survive.

Foreword

■ A Word from the Author/Acknowledgement

Since the fall of 1997, as author of six college textbooks, I proved to students (and myself) how *applied psychology* enriches a variety of societal contexts. Two texts dedicated to the workplace, *Cognitive Strategies: Psychology in the Workplace* and *Interpersonal Psychology: Communicating Effective People Skills* put psychology to "work" with an introduction to cognitive psych and industrial/organizational psych.

In the classroom, an introductory text *Psychology: Brain, Behavior, and Popular Culture* gave students an eclectic survey of the methodologies and perspectives of psychology as a behavioral science amid existential pop culture. "At risk" students and students already on academic probation were shown the relationship between the "hard-wired" brilliance of the brain, becoming smarter in the college experience, and cover-all-bases adjustment strategies with *Psychology of Adjustment: Surviving the College Experience*.

In clinical psychology *Inside the Clinical Picture* allowed students entry beyond the waiting room of clinical practice to disclose what really happens between client and clinician with the myriad of issues in overcoming psychopathology.

Along the way, my son Nick Jacobs and I collaborated on the novel *Freak Accident,* to demonstrate how a novel of fiction can use metaphor to apply to the higher expectations of the college experience. The WC freshman class of 2002 wrote some startling essay to prove students are not "going to the dogs," although they may be "going to the wolves"! You're going to have to read *Freak Accident* to figure that one out.

In Spring 2003, I decided to break new ground on a subject I thought to be fascinating, but due to the profundity of subject matter, frankly, I felt a little intimidated. Through the years I kept telling myself I knew just enough about serial killers to satisfy my intellectual curiosity and that was enough. What more could I possible need to know about Ted Bundy, Jeffery Dahmer, and the human predators known as serial rapists and killers? After all, there's plenty of programming on the subject courtesy of *Court TV.*

Perhaps, I feared peering too deeply into the abyss of human depravity as Robert Ressler warned in *Whoever Fights Monsters.* Too, I was aware of the psychological "meltdown" experienced by ex-FBI profiler, John Douglas recounted in *Journey into Darkness.* As always, when "push came to shove," students convinced me the book *had to be written.* I seldom argue with students, especially when they ask compelling questions. What factors lie behind psychopathy? What makes serial killers tick?

The text you hold in your hands offers an introduction to *psychopathic personality,* specifically the dangerous *sexual psychopaths* who become serial killers—the true monsters of society. Along the way, we will investigate psychological principles underlying the study of psychopathy as well as the "mousetrap"—the criminal profile—used to catch them. The journey of writing a textbook is both a stimulating and exhausting adventure, and in this case, an impossible task without my criminal profiling students and teaching assistants (in our lingo "PAs," or psych teaching assistants) who were beside me all the way.

The sixteen weeks of spring semester 2003 were spent in chapter development. Insights from our research were both shocking and, at times, gut wrenching. At some points I felt my reach had exceeded my grasp. I wondered if my students were mature enough to handle the impact of the material. Privately, I wondered if I was! To me, the experience reflected the values of higher education—experiences that are life changing, liberating, insightful, maturing, and ultimately, in this case, cautionary. In today's world, we are all "behavioral scientists" whether or not we care to be. Accurately "reading" the behavior of others may save our life. Living amid existential reality—living in a world fraught with modern problems—we better know who we are dealing with.

Tangentially, this book is about loving nurturing parenting and the children it produces versus the antithesis—hateful antisocial parenting—and the monsters it produces.

As it turns out, the true monsters of society are the abusive and hateful parents who are incompetent, chemically addicted, emotionally inaccessible, and unloving, who raise emotionally bruised children heading straight into sexual psychopathy. Those with the most physical and emotional trauma suffer irreversible neurological damage and become sexual psychopaths—serial killers.

The human spirit may soar at times, but it can fall down into the basement of unspeakable depravity, transforming the very essence of innocence into a disgusting reptilian mind hiding behind a human face.

Below, my inaugural criminal profiling students are listed by name. As a whole, they contributed mightily to this project, a project that started approximately three years ago when I first started my cluttered "mental file" by slowly gathering resources, reading every book I could find on psychopathy, and deciding how to present the subject in an engaging way.

It is my honor to recognize all thirty-seven students (and seven magnificent **PAs**—my indispensable psych teaching assistants) for providing a therapeutic milieu for a worthwhile writing adventure. All of us hope all of you will enjoy the insights as much as we enjoyed bringing them to light.

Very special thanks to Valerie Warren, PA, and Rae Ellen Wooten, PA, for editing selected chapters. Special thanks to Mary Pike for editing the entire manuscript. Thanks to my editor David Pike, and Billee Jo Hefel, and the gang at Kendall/Hunt for technical and marketing support.

◼ Criminal Profiling Class of Spring 2003

Stacy Arnett
Jackie Arwood
Jeffrey Barker
Anna Boswell
Kimberly Bunt
Jeremy Carter
Amber Coffee
Jennifer Coffee
Wanda Cox
Jeremy Crabb
Mary Ellis
Kieran Evans
Sandra Forrester
Amanda Frank
Derek Gibson
Erica Grisham
Jeremy Harrison
Megan Henn
Michelle Heins, PA
Lauren Hughes
Meagan Hurst
Brenda Jaime
Heather Kidd
Blaine Kosikowski

Faie Lafleur
Heather Marshall
Daniel McCarty
Brandon McGinnis
Michelle Mejia
Heather Mitchell, PA
Clarissa Noland
Nia Nolan
Sara Reynolds
Ashley Richardson, PA
Amanda Roderick
Chris Rutledge
Brettne Sanders, PA
Jack Shannon
Brett Shayler, PA
Kenneth Strickland
Neil Tilly
Sonia Todd
Shawn Vandercook
Valeria Warren, PA
Chasidy Wilson
Amanda Woolsey
Rae Ellen Wooten, PA

■ Organization Matters

In the simplest terms, this book is divided into eight chapters with two *Predator Profiles*—bios of serial killers—in each chapter, except for chapter eight. When a word or expression is in **bold type** it is defined in the **Word Scholar Glossary** in the addendum as important technical or scholarly words. To obtain a clear understanding of the word, students should stop, mark their place in the chapter, and proceed directly to the glossary for the definition of the word. In contrast, when a word or expression is stressed for importance, it is *italicized* and does not appear in the glossary.

A special kind of "running" commentary exists for reader-author interaction via email at anytime. Readers may email author Don Jacobs at *djacobs@wc.edu* to make observations, comments, suggestions, or to ask questions regarding the content of the book.

CHAPTER 1

The Sexual Psychopath: Psychopathy & Serial Crime

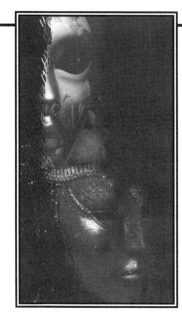

66 *. . . Police learned another thing the killer did: Bill kept them for a while, alive. These victims didn't die until a week to ten days after they were abducted . . . he had to have a place to keep them and a place to work in privacy. It meant he wasn't a drifter. He was more of a trapdoor spider . . .* **99**

—*Silence of the Lambs*
Thomas Harris

Psychopathic personality: an emotionally and behaviorally disordered state characterized by *clear perception of reality* except for the individual's social and moral obligations, and often by the *pursuit of immediate personal gratification in criminal acts, drug addiction, or sexual perversion.*

—Webster's Collegiate Dictionary (10 Ed.)

■ View to a Kill

In 1998, twenty-one year old Donta (Don-Tay) Page, living in a halfway house and after spending the night on the streets, followed a young woman to her home. When the woman, twenty-four year old Peyton Tuthill, left her apartment again for a job interview, Page broke into her apartment to steal something to sell. On her return, she surprised him. A fierce physical battle ensued. After he subdued her, he tied her hands and arms with an electrical cord. Then he left, but changed his mind and returned.

When she saw him, she cried and begged for her life. He slit her throat to stop her screams. He cut her hands and wrists to stop her from fighting. Then, he stabbed her repeatedly until he killed her. Upon his arrest after the murder, he confessed to the horrific crime.

According to forensic psychiatrist Dr. Dorothy O. Lewis (*Guilty By Reason of Insanity*), Donta Page was a "walking textbook" in the clinical evaluation of severe child abuse. As a child, his mother physically abused him repeatedly. As early as first grade he was markedly withdrawn. By second grade, a mental health examination was ordered due to his inactivity in the classroom. By age ten, medical records showed he had been repeatedly **sodomized**. Warnings—"red flags" of psychopathy—were everywhere. He so desperately needed intervention and treatment by a caring adult, but received none.

According to neurologist John Pincus, *violent criminals* have extensive prefrontal lobe damage. Neuroscientist Adrian Raine of UCLA performed a brain scan of Donta Page's prefrontal cortex and results showed minimal functioning. Page's brain was "cool-coded," showing decreased prefrontal cerebral activity (observed in scarcity of blood flow, glowing blue in the scan, hence "cool-coded").

Can severe brain damage to prefrontal lobes—the seat of restraint and strategic thinking related to behavioral consequence—unleash violent behavior on unsuspecting victims? The intrusion of *forensic neuroscience* into the courtroom—clinical neuropsychologists showing "cool-coded" brain scans of killers to curious jurors—in the past decade has been startling. Yet, not everyone is duly impressed with expert witnesses spouting "neuro-psychobabble" and showing off "cool-coded" brain scans, as if they were forensic trophies. For example, Dr. Dan Martell, a forensic neuropsychologist, believes neuroscience is overused in the courtroom. According to Dr. Martell, "brain damage itself is not the root cause of crime; it depends on the case and the situation."

Peyton Tuthill's mother believes Donta Page murdered her daughter because "he is evil."

With neuroscience firmly in the middle of the courtroom and on the minds of the jurors, would Donta Page's documented brain damage save him from lethal injection? At the end of the trial, jurors returned a verdict of "guilty on all counts". Subsequently, the trial judge sentenced Page to life without parole. In this case, the defense of prefrontal neurological damage mitigating first-degree murder worked. As frustrated criminal prosecutors will tell you, the defense of "cool-coded" brain scans "hits" more often than it "misses".

■ Innocence Destroyed

In 1995, twenty-three year old Jeremy Skocz (Scotch) committed a vicious and inhuman crime. He murdered a four year old child. In childhood, Skocz spent five horrific years with heroin-addicted parents who were convicted felons. They never attempted to hide their antisocial lifestyle from their son. Everyday, he lived amid hateful, unloving, and drug-**addled** parenting.

When Skocz was seven years old, he was adopted into a healthy family milieu. The family, in his words, was almost "too perfect". Everything seemed to turn around for the young boy, but something happened. When he was fifteen years old, walking home through a park, he was attacked by an assailant with a baseball bat and violently hit in the face and head. With an already damaged brain from the emotional backlash of antisocial parenting, the head trauma permanently and radically *changed his personality*. In the coming weeks he became increasingly withdrawn and brooding.

Without warning, Skocz left the safety of his adopted home to find his birth father. He found him in his house trailer smoking a joint. Nothing had changed. Nevertheless, Scotz remained with his birth father. Soon, he started using hard drugs. Although he looked normal, he was barely keeping the lid on his growing rage, frustration, and disappointment for being "different" and for feeling abandoned by his birth parents.

The Cox family lived next door to Jeremy's birth father. One evening near dusk, four year old Shelby Cox disappeared from her front porch. Worried, her parents quickly formed a search party. Jeremy volunteered in the search. In a shocking surprise, Skocz led authorities directly to the shed were he hid her body.

Criminal investigation showed he bound her with duct tape to prevent her from running away, and raped her twice while he suffocated her to death with duct tape. He stuffed her small body into a garbage bag, covered it with a gym bag, and stuffed her body like trash into a cabinet.

In prison when asked by an investigator "Why did you kill her?" Skotz replied, "I don't know." After a long pause he continued, "I can't answer that question."

■ "Cool-Coded" Brain Scans

After the murder, a series of neurological brain scans were run on Skotz showing the same pattern of "cool-coded" prefrontal lobe damage. Due to the emotional abyss of antisocial parenting, the attack on his head from the baseball bat, and the use of hard drugs in attempting to self-medicate, Skotz's brain was severely and irreparably "fractured". A forensic psychologist testified, "Skotz lived in a broken body."

The jury accepted evidence of brain damage mitigating cognitive premeditation required for first-degree murder so that Jeremy Skotz will spend the rest of his life in prison, signaling another "victory" for neuroscience in the courtroom. Apparently, juries are no longer "blinded by science", they are, in fact, embracing it.

Although Donta Page and Jeremy Skotz were not serial killers, would they have become serial predators if not for their capture and subsequent incarceration? The same question will be posed in Chapter Seven for adolescent "Rambo" killers who kill classmates and adults in home and schoolplace violence. Before we look closer, let's explore a short history lesson in folklore by addressing the world's first serial killers.

■ Folklore—The First Serial Killers

Obscured by centuries, displaced by time and **zeitgeist**, far from the modern practice of criminal profiling are instances of society's first serial killers. In the sixteenth and seventeenth centuries in rural areas of France and

Germany, vicious, apparently motiveless murders were discovered along country roads and pastureland. Sometimes weekly, farmers discovered bodies of mutilated children and adults. As the body count steadily rose, fear turned to outrage. Hunting parties were formed to track the vile predators, but without modern profiling what did the crime scene disclose? What about the physical characteristics of the predator? What was his motivation? More, importantly, what did he look like? What did villagers have to go on other than bloodhounds and anger?

Remarkably, vicious human-wolves were targeted as the world's first serial killers. Deranged human males became snarling, "devil-spawned" werewolves referred to as "lycanthropes," (from the word **lycanthropy**, a modern psychiatric condition characterized by patients who imagine they are wolves. They may howl at the moon, run around on all fours, and imagine a heightened sense of smell.) The lycanthropes (like-en-throps), documented by historical records, savagely attacked victims, tearing them to shreds. They repeated their crimes in sequential fashion with a period of inactivity (the "cooling off" period observed in serial homicide).

Apparently, some lycanthropes were able to alter their appearance with wolfen characteristics such as growing facial hair and by filing their teeth to a sharp, canine point. A French hermit, Gilles Garnier, stalked and killed numerous children, and then cannibalized their corpses.

Stalked like an animal himself by angry villagers, Garnier was captured and burned alive at the stake as a werewolf in 1573, thus preventing further instances of serial murder.

Over a twenty-five year period, another werewolf, Peter Stubbe, terrorized adults and children as a serial killer around Cologne, Germany in the sixteenth century. According to records, Stubbe could change his shape (hence the term "shape shifting" in werewolf literature) displaying . . "eyes great and large, which in the night sparkled like brands of fire; mouth great and wide, with sharp and cruel teeth, a huge body and mighty claws." (Everitt).

Like Garnier, Stubbe stalked his prey and staged a bloody, savage attack just like real wolves attacking prey. In another practice reflecting his deranged mind, Stubbe repeatedly committed incest with his own daughter and "recruited" her to help him lure unsuspecting victims. The abusive manipulator and his compliant daughter provided one of the first instances of a *compliant co-offender.*

Stubbe was hunted and eventually captured. He was executed in the following way: "strapped to a wheel, ten hot pincers were used to tear away his flesh in ten places, then his arms and legs were crushed with the head of an axe, his head decapitated and his body burned. His decapitated head was put on the top of a pole bearing the picture of a wolf." (Everitt) In our "enlightened" society, convicted serial rapists and murderers—modern werewolves—sit on death row for approximately ten years on average, eat three hot meals a day, and receive free medical and dental attention. Victim advocacy groups ask "why?"

The fear of wolves killing children and livestock in rural areas may have influenced the perception of wolfen characteristics to the unkempt appearance of both Garnier and Stubbe. In all probably, the vile killers suffered from psychotic delusions and imagined themselves as demonic wolves. It is true that wolves, in fact all wild animals, are serial killers—they kill sequentially as a mere act of survival; only human predators, serial killers, derive *emotional* and *sexual thrills* from controlling another person and deciding when they die.

Analyzed by modern psychiatric criteria, Garnier and Stubbe would be likely diagnosed with psychosis driven by sexual obsessions; an alternative diagnosis of paranoid schizophrenia might apply. Today, experts know that *most serial killers are not psychotic;* they know exactly what they're doing, and that's the scary part.

The study of *modern serial homicide began in the nineteenth century* with the murders of prostitutes by Jack the Ripper in 1888. Both the appearance of serial killers and the methods of punishment (electrocution, lethal gas, lethal injection) have changed drastically.

◼ Beyond Folklore—Today's Existential Reality

Today, serial killers remain partially human, mostly animal. He rapes and murders mostly strangers, not for survival, but for **macabre** fascination and compulsive desire to control life and death in an unsuspecting victim. Controlling, manipulating, and dominating an unsuspecting victim marks the only control he has ever experienced in his otherwise aimless life. In our nomenclature, his behavior is termed **rapacious**—he is a sexual psychopath who preys upon victims for the "thrilling high" of perverted sexual self-gratification. To the world he is known as a serial rapist or serial killer. He rapes and murders for sexual control, domination, degradation, and perhaps worst of *all, sexual experimentation.* And, he will never stop. Upon capture, he must be incarcerated for life without parole, or be put to death by lethal injection. There exists no treatment or therapy to reverse sexual psychopathy.

He is likely frustrated and angry from the effects of hateful antisocial parenting, but he has found a way to channel his rage for being "different". He lives in a scary, inner world where every aspect of rape and/or killing is *sexualized*—to the last detail. Plain and simple, *he is a sexual deviant and a sexual predator.* Most assuredly, he is a sexual addict. He may be a religious fanatic or an antheistic nihilist. He may be a paranoid schizophrenic, though seldom is he psychotic. Although neurologically damaged, he knows he is a predator.

He will never be anything more than a cowardly, pathetic loser who preys upon unsuspecting victims for sexual gratification—a "gratification" that is ultimately non-fulfilling in the sense of impassioned lovers fulfilling each other's emotional and sexual needs. He is addicted to the "high" of his own brain chemistry. He feels "compelled" to continue by the unrelenting "brutal urge." Soon, he is out searching for another victim.

Just as no one wakes up one morning and "decides" to become a serial killer, **antecedent** events from his horrific childhood prevent him from ever enjoying a normal life. Sexual predators' abusive history comes from antisocial parenting, addiction to pornography and/or deviant websites, perverted cognitive mapping, or sexual repression from a hateful and domineering mother.

He prowls under any moon and may strike in broad daylight on a busy street. He's cunning, deliberate, and increasingly arrogant. In his **narcissism**, he feels much smarter than those who pursue him. His victims don't know him, but according to notorious serial killer Ted Bundy, the organized offender "knows his subjects very well". Often, he visits them in dreams or anywhere else in society he desires. He chooses the time and the place. Finally, he's found something he can control. He bets his victims are naïve and unsuspecting. He wagers they never thought it would happen to them. He catches them off guard and completely unaware.

He stalks his victims from afar and now he's near. With the mind of an addict and the face of a human masking a reptile, he's the modern version of the werewolf profiled as a serial rapist or serial killer. Perhaps as many as 50 or more at any given time are on the prowl in North America alone and his numbers are growing and changing.

◼ Now . . . and Then

The young musical artist raises the microphone to his lips in the semi-dark studio. The words of a well known song about "not letting life pass you by" merges with musical accompaniment. Heads and faces of audience members are barely seen as they sing along with the well-known words. Band members move around the stage as only musicians move to the cadence of music. The studio comes alive with movement and rhythm. The singer is Brandon Boyd. The song is "Warning" by the alternative rock group *Incubus*. The year is 2003.

In another place and another time, the singer in the studio could have been Charles Manson. Like Boyd, he loved music. He loved to sing. He loved to play the guitar. He associated with other musicians such as Dennis Wilson of the *Beach Boys*. He envisioned rock star status. The year was 1969.

For certain, Brandon Boyd, creative force behind his group, and Charles Manson, incarcerated "mastermind" of murder, are galaxies apart. Yet, similarities are interesting. Boyd is charismatic and engaging to his audience; he writes his own music. Today, many journalists who have interviewed Manson contend that he remains charismatic to a new generation. He still writes his own music. Manson was responsible, more than any other person, for bringing worldwide attention to the word "psychopathic" due to his brainwashed teenagers, judged ultimately responsible for the Tate-LaBianca murders. The Manson Family (subjects of Predator Profile 7-2 in Chapter Seven) received infamous fame for two separate crimes occurring in Los Angeles, California in 1969.

Crushed by failure, Manson became bitter when his dream of a recording contract never materialized. One is an accomplished artist, the other a failed manipulator. Boyd is wealthy and free to move about society. He recently recorded "The Morning View Sessions," a new CD, in a California mansion. Manson is incarcerated for life and resides in a California prison. Boyd has tattoos. Manson has a swastika carved on his forehead right between his eyes.

Boyd respects and nurtures life through his music; Manson disrespected life and in his paranoid view of the world saw a nihilistic society heading into "Helter Skelter"—an out-of-control race war. Manson preyed upon others and took everything from them—their lives—accomplished by his brainwashed teenage "family". The crime scenes must have been shocking. The victims never saw it coming in the hot August nights of Southern California.

Had Manson persisted in his musical dreams he might have succeeded. "The Manson Family" might have referred to his backup group instead of his mind-controlled murderers, who will spend the remaining years of their lives in prison. Boyd—a creator, Manson—a destroyer. Both are artists who took different paths. Why?

Sexual Predators: Serial Killers in the Age of Neuroscience is an attempt to collect pieces of the puzzle. What does behavioral science and neuropsychology know about the development of sexual psychopaths? In the process, how does the "mousetrap"—the criminal profile—aid law enforcement in catching this perverted and elusive predator?

◼ Sexual Psychopathy

Clinically, **serial killers** are diagnosed with antisocial personality. Yet, the clinical definition of antisocial personality disorder, when compared to the *profundity of pathology* and the *sexual perversity* inherent in serial crime, simply does not adequately describe the *deviance* of this disgusting monster hiding behind a human face.

According to the *DSM (Diagnostic and Statistical Manual of Mental Disorders)*, the clinical reference book used by clinical psychologists and psychiatrists, the diagnostic feature of the **Antisocial Personality Disorder** is a pervasive pattern of disregard for, and violation of, the rights of others that begins in childhood or early adolescence and continues into adulthood. The DSM version of a sexually perverted, criminal personality is far too antiseptic and clinical to portray the macabre perversion of sexual psychopathy in the guise of serial killers and rapists.

While serial killers certainly fit antisocial pathology, the true nature of their heinous acts—*behaviorally and emotionally*—reaches far down into the "crawlspace" of human depravity. Deviance beyond human rationality—the sanctum of **sexual psychopathy**—succinctly describes the depraved mind and sexualized crimes of serial killers. Plain and simple, serial killers are sexual psychopaths—sexual deviants with no remorse, no conscience. Once captured, there is no treatment. *Sexual psychopaths are sexual deviants for life.*

◼ Adolescent "Rambo" Killers

Some children not yet old enough to drive are making up a growing list of kids too young to qualify as serial predators, but nonetheless, they are "kids who kill kids and adults" in homeplace and schoolplace violence—adolescent "Rambo" killers—in our nomenclature. *They often target the face of victims.* Due to the current *zeitgeist,* in 1998 the FBI felt compelled to publish the first ever *schoolplace violence profile* (contained in Chapter Six).

This book is about the psychosocial, familial, developmental, and startling neurological evidence from brain scanning technology disclosing the mind of serial killers. Tangentially, the book addresses the "mousetrap"—the criminal profile—the investigative document meticulously prepared by profilers intent upon catching human predators walking around in civilized society in the camouflage of neighbors, friends, and co-workers.

◼ The Atlanta Murders

First Test of Profiling

Is the "profile" a viable investigative tool or mere "hocus pocus"? The *art and science* of criminal profiling first came under the harsh glare of media and public scrutiny when it claimed center stage in the high profile murders of many black youths in Atlanta, Georgia. In the summer of 1981, the FBI Academy at Quantico, Virginia sent FBI profilers John Douglas and Roy Hazelwood to Atlanta to test the controversial tool resting on the principle that crime scene date and victimology could "narrow down" the search to one suspect, using principles of psychology, common sense, good luck, and timing. Unknown to the general public, the FBI had an ace up their sleeve—*known offender characteristics of serial killers*—in a recently created FBI database.

Police officers working the case were skeptical as were many agents within the FBI. How could "a profile" be worth the paper it was written on? How could knowledge of psychology disclose probable behavior and personality of rapists and killers?

Using speculative logic, common sense (something Sherlock Holmes was famous for), principles of psychology, and a database of *known offender characteristics* gathered years earlier by interviewing incarcerated serial criminals, Douglas and Hazelwood created a criminal profile. The profile fit the offender Wayne Williams with such uncanny accuracy that all doubters were silenced. The document suggested the offender was a young black male and a police "buff," who impersonated police officers. This **ruse** allowed the *UNSUB* (the unidentified subject, in FBI lingo) ready access to his young, unsuspecting victims. The profile was so accurate observers commented "it was as though the agents were watching the killer's every move even when he committed the murders and dumped the bodies".

During the trail, Douglas predicted Williams would fain a heart attack in court when the tide of evidence turned against him. He did. He suggested a strategy in interrogating Williams on the witness stand that might trigger the rage Williams hid under his carefully crafted persona. During questioning, Douglas instructed the prosecuting attorney to invade his personal space, grab Williams' hands and in a low, barely audible voice, inches from his face, ask "What was it like to wrap your fingers around your victims' throats? Were you frightened?" Shocked, Williams replied "No." Realizing what he had done, Williams angrily jumped from his seat blasting the attorney "you're not going to implicate me with your profile"!

To actually experience this outburst of rage in the middle of the proceedings (along with forensic evidence—hair and fiber samples gathered at the crime scene—matching evidence in Williams' home) the jury was convinced. They convicted Wayne Williams of the Atlanta child murders and sent him to prison for life. Williams maintains his innocence to this day.

■ Psychology & Criminal Profiling

Before analyzing the mind of a *special category of killers* with psychopathic personality emblazoned with sexual psychopathy—*serial killers*—we first address an important question. Could there be accurate profiling without underlying psychological principles? The answer is clearly "no."

Admittedly, a very rudimentary kind of criminal overview, borrowing from criminology, sociology, and criminal justice, might offer a crude sketch of a perpetrator based on crime trends, statistics, and criminal typologies; however, the document would be devoid of significant and important pieces of the puzzle—the *emotional* and *sexual* components, and the *behavioral habits* and *patterns* characteristic of sexual psychopathy. It appears that emotional factors—the **affective** (feeling) component of the human mind—dominate the **cognitive** (thinking) component fueling perverted sexual desire.

In the early 1990s, the key ingredients of profiling—psychological, emotional, and behavioral—comprised the profile's first media moniker, known as the *psycho-behavioral profile*. By the same moniker, it was mentioned in *The Silence of the Lambs,* the Academy Awards® Best Picture of 1992. Today, it is simply known as "the profile".

Without psychological principles, the mind of a violent criminal capable of *rapacious behavior—behavior that preys upon others in sexualized ways*—could not be analyzed in-depth.

The mission of this book is not to be a primer or a tutorial on the ways and means of writing a criminal profile. At the end of the day, readers will not be qualified to offer services to law enforcement agencies as an independent profiler. Nor should they. According to the ex-FBI special agents and modern founders of criminal profiling (Robert Ressler, John Douglas, Roy Hazelwood, and others), it takes years of training, expertise, research, maturity, and experience to author effective profiles. (Common sense and luck are also helpful, they note.)

◼ Criminal Diagnosticians

Profiler John Douglas cautions law enforcement personnel on the dangers of becoming a profiler by attending a three-day seminar or by mail order. Competent profilers seek to "enter the mind" of criminals as *criminal diagnosticians* to discover tendencies, proclivities, fantasies, habits, and lifestyle. In the process, profilers learn how vulnerable the serial killer is in being apprehended, as all criminals leave considerable information about themselves behind at the crime scene.

The behavior of serial predators "chatter" at the crime scene, leaving important clues about his crimes to those skilled enough to notice. When criminal investigators arrive at a crime scene the chase is on.

◼ Antisocial Parenting

The scary, sexualized, inner world of sexual predators and the documented psychological, social, behavioral, and neurochemical influences that shape human monsters, demonstrates the devastation of abusive and loveless parenting—**antisocial parenting**. This netherworld of toxic parenting along with other "root" causes, provides the demonic "recipe" for creating a child with a *psychopathic personality delineated by sexual psychopathy.*

We have answers from neuroscience, theory, and speculative logic— the investigative and theoretical tools of behavioral science. Readers and students of forensic psychology and violent criminal investigation will be permitted to peer deep inside the mind of serial predators. What is discovered is terrifying. Usually, *neurological devastation is so extensive* it is displayed in sophisticated brain scanning devices. Therefore, no therapeutic treatment, no "talk therapy" will ever be effective. Nothing currently available in neuroscience or clinical neuropsychology works to help sexual psychopaths "recover". (Yet, Chapter Eight provides a prescient look into what some consider a viable alternative to non-existent treatment that may be only years away.)

What readers will know after reading this text is how a human infant with so much promise and expectation of living a full, normal life, surrounded by loving family, friends, and a productive career can be psychologically "disfigured" and "reduced" to a repulsive reptile on the prowl for human prey to rape and/or murder.

Criminal profilers agree that all *serial killers* are sexually perverted and they behave irrationally.

◼ Abbreviated Psychopathy Checklist

The recognized authority on psychopathy, Robert Hare, Ph.D., produced, along with his colleagues and students, *The Hare Psychopathy Checklist-Revised (PCL-R),* an instrument used to determine characteristics of psychopathic personality. The most recognizable characteristic of psychopathy include individuals who have a gift of *engaging others.* We have modified and condensed Hare's original psychopathy list to twenty characteristics in no particular order. The garden variety psychopath (in our nomenclature) may not be a sexual psychopath—a serial killer. While gender is irrelevant in *garden variety psychopathy,* males often display features of **narcissism**, while females display **histrionic** features. Both genders may populate business, industry, education, and the clergy as successful community leaders.

A "cookie-cutter" example of this type of "white collar" psychopathy recently gained notoriety as individuals who were corporate heads of *World.Com* and *Enron.* Playboy magazine, a longtime harbinger of pop culture hedonism, provided a reminder of the seductive allure of psychopathy in a pictorial display of ex-Enron female employees. Less recently, a famous football hero fit the same profile of narcissism mixed with psychopathy and was held civilly responsible for the deaths of his ex-wife and her friend. According to former LA prosecutor, Vincent Bugilosi, O.J. Simpson has not found the murderer he pledged to find, even as he searches in vain for the killer on golf courses where he spends most of his time.

The *garden variety psychopath* displays:

1. Grandiose sense of self-worth
2. Glib, superficial charm
3. Need for stimulation; prone to boredom
4. Lack of remorse or guilt (including criminal behavior)
5. Pathological liar
6. Callous, lack of empathy for others
7. Perhaps charismatic, certainly engaging to most individuals
8. Shallow emotional response, blunt affect (lack of facial expression)
9. Parasitic lifestyle
10. Sexual promiscuity
11. Impulsive
12. Lack of realistic long-term goals
13. Poor behavioral controls (lack of restraint in getting what they want)
14. Early behavioral problems (conduct disorders, oppositional defiance)
15. Irresponsible
16. Failure to accept responsibility for actions (deflection of responsibility)
17. Many short-term relationships; never accepts blame for termination of relationships
18. Juvenile delinquency
19. Criminal versatility
20. Cunning and manipulative

Interestingly, there are no *clinical diagnostic criteria* for psychopathy in the DSM. The word "psychopathy" or "psychopathic personality" is not found in the DSM index.

Denotatively, a **psychopath** (a person with *psychopathic personality features*) is not technically the same individual with a diagnosis of antisocial personality disorder (which is listed in the clusters of personality disorders in the DSM). However, connotatively, the two terms have merged into one in general usage. Although serial killers are diagnosed with antisocial personality disorder, they are more accurately **sexual psychopaths**—human predators that rape and kill others for the *emotional "high"* of sexual control and domination. In most cases, the majority of serial killers experiment sexually with their victims as sexual "lab specimens."

Psychopaths display a *pronounced inability to feel emotionally connected to anyone except as a source of sexual stimulation.*

While sexual psychopaths possess a psychopathic personality—emotional and behavioral state characterized by *clear perception of reality* except for perversity of social and moral obligations, they pursue immediate personal gratification in criminal acts, drug addiction, and sexual perversion. The clearest delineation we offer for this special type of criminal is: *serial killers are sexual deviants with psychopathic personalities delineated by sexual psychopathy.*

Hare (*Without Conscience*) discovered that criminal psychopaths contain over 30 or more psychopathic traits in his *psychopathy checklist* (out of a possible 40). Imagine how many "lesser" psychopaths (with lower scores) roam freely in society and have never been arrested, much less incarcerated. Nonetheless, they damage almost everyone they touch in emotional ways that linger long after the psychopath seeks greener pastures.

◼ Camouflaged Psychopaths

Realistically, some highly functional psychopaths are camouflaged in various societal venues—sports, business, politics, arts, religion, and education. Psychopathic individuals litter pop culture. They may be current or retired sports heroes, business executives, politicians, and Hollywood artisans and agents. Some celebrity psychopaths have been tried for murder or for hiring a hit man to kill a wife or girlfriend. Finally, they may hide in the ivory towers of education, the only category not affiliated with pop culture, yet populated with garden variety psychopathy in blissful anonymity, causing emotional upheaval in underlings and students.

This book is not about the thousands, perhaps millions of psychopathic individuals who "terrorize" others in the workplace by analyzing the power structure of the organization and aligning themselves with authority. They are astute observers of human behavior as they plot the downfall of "competitors" in such crafty ways that almost no one suspects them.

Interestingly, functional non-criminal psychopathy—below the violent criminal variety of murderers, serial rapists, and serial killers—may actually be advantageous in business and industry. Consider for a moment all the superficially glib, compulsive lying, "stab you in the back" narcissists you have known. Perhaps you currently work alongside such individuals. "Psychopaths in business suits" are what some experts refer to as functional, non-criminal psychopaths.

The difference between the non-criminal types and the serial killer variety is the *profundity* of familial abuse, addiction to hardcore pornography, the deviancy of cognitive mapping, and most importantly, the presence of severe, irreversible neurological damage to specific brain areas.

What Lies Beneath—A Social Commentary
of Psychopathic Proportions

The profundity of inexcusable behavior on the part of former Baylor University basketball coach Dave Bliss both *pre* and *post* the sad disappearance and death of Patrick Dennehy and the entire fiasco that once resembled a college basketball program was, in a way, predictable. Yes, predictable. Even after a thirty-year charade. Psychology has come a long way beyond Thunderdome and psychobabble. Welcome to the age of cognitive and behavioral neuroscience.

The train wreck waiting to happen just needed the right conditions—in Coach Bliss's words albeit—"bizarre" conditions. And, it took thirty years. But, cracks in his ethical foundation had been visible even in his career at other colleges. According to behavioral psychology—the same psychology that underlies the FBI's success with criminal profiling—all any of us have to do in "figuring out" another person is just watch behavior. Watch it *very carefully:* not for surface shine but for *what lies beneath.* An armchair will do, you don't need a Ph.D. in clinical forensic psychology. The behavior we're talking about is "right in your face" behavior. Predictably, it will be nothing more than persona. We all know why the Phantom of the Opera wore a mask. He was hiding something. Yet, his disfigurement was apparaent long before the unmasking.

What lies beneath persona (Carl Jung's term for a person's camouflage or "social mask") is the real deal—call it naked character. At the least, persona is misleading, and at most it is "telling." Why? Because behavior (including camouflaged persona) speaks volumes to those skilled enough to notice that *behavior discloses personality, even what lie beneath layers of camouflage.* Personality is multi-dimensional and yes, reflective of customary habits and patterns of behavior. But, personality is also a façade for the "print" (like a fingerprint) of character (maverick personality theorist Freud preferred the word character to the word personality).

For scores of athletes, former sports icons, coaches, athletic directors, actors, business leaders, politicians, and any and all high profile professions heavy into public relations where image is tony—complications from *psychopathic personality* is the train wreck waiting to happen. Dave Bliss is no different than a score of others who admitted infidelities such as O.J. Simpson, Kobe Bryant, Mike Tyson, Scott Peterson, or anyone else who has committed *morally* despicable acts worthy of the evening news. From a psychological perspective, Bliss is not "bad" or "evil." What Bliss, and a long list of others in sports and business are displaying, is behavioral *psychopathy,* plain and simple. Psychopathic behavior translates to *not really caring about other people.* Not really. Except for sexual stimulation, novelty, praise, publicity, and/or monetary gain, that is. Of course, when psychopaths get caught, they sing a different tune and appear repentant. They're really sorry . . . sorry they got caught. They didn't make a silly human mistake either (because they're much too cunning for that).

(continues)

(continued)

They knew exactly what they were doing and they're betting others are too stupid, too adoring, or too fanatical (as in sports "fan," the shorthand version) to ever suspect them. And, here's a news flash—they'll keep doing it. And, most people never see it coming . . . they never see *what lies beneath.*

Phillipe Pinel, the nineteenth century founder of French psychiatry, observed a distrubing behavior in some patients that spelled trouble for everyone who crossed their path long enough to have "dealings." He termed the character disorder *manie sans delire* or "obsessive behavior without insanity." The *DSM (Diagnostic and Statistical Manual of Mental Disorders)* echoed Pinel's taxonomy with diagnostic criteria for psychopathy with a lame version, *antisocial personality disorder.* Take heed taskforce advisors of the APA, the criteria doesn't come close to characterizing the specificity or profundity of psychopathy for a bird with the cognitive and behavioral characteristics of Bliss and scores like him. A common dictionary definition is better. According to *Webster's Collegiate,* psychopathic personality is an emotionally and behaviorally disordered state characterized by *clear perception of reality* except for the individual's *social and moral obligations,* and often by the *pursuit of immediate personal gratification in criminal acts,* drug addition, or sexual perversion.

Essentially, psychopathy *denotes a continuum of severity* from "mild" to "severe" outwardly camouflaged with socially desirable, even celebrated behavior. Yet, what lies beneath the glib (slippery), superficial "gentlemanly" charm, is a deeper pathology characterized by lack of emotional attachment, insincerity, compulsive lying, and at the core of all "social" psychopaths—lack of empathy for other people and their troubles, *schadenfreude,* dishonesty or fabrication of events, and failure to own up for moral ineptitude ("I did not have sex with that intern!"). Hubris aside, we don't need Freud to make a diagnosis of psychopathic personality—*psychopathy* is the common cold of pop culture USA hedonism—seeking pleasure at the expense of others because it's fun, stimulating, and powerful, driven largely by NOS libido. (This explains why, in some individuals, "mild" to "moderate" psychopathy lessens with age.)

To clinicians, psychopathy runs along a behavioral continuum from "mild" to "moderate" versions (which are usually non-criminal) to "severe" criminal varieties. In males, "mild" to "moderate" varieties of psychopathy when mixed with a dose of narissism and camera friendly looks, produces an O.J. Simpson clone or a Bill Clinton clone. In business and industry, we have many instances of "psychopaths in suits" with Enron and World.com executives displaying core psychopathy—lack of empathy and genuine concern for others, and failure to take responsiblity or ultimate blame for blatant "white-collar" criminality. Like adolescents with raging hormones, psychopaths feel bulletproof due in part to intoxicated self-importance. Moderate to severe psychopathy comes dangerously close to Nietzsche's idea of the Superman cinematically presented in Alfred Hitchcock's *Rope.*

(continues)

(continued)

In the camouflage of business, athletics, sports, and politics, "mild" to "moderate" psychopathy may, *in persona,* produce a very likeable, personally engaging, and charismatic person. He fools people day in and day out because . . . well he's so believable and he's such a nice guy. Yet, what lies beneath the snake charmer is a reptilian viper. Enter neuroscience and brain scans. In severe psychopathy, the reptilian brain (the brain stem) and mid-brain ("old mammalian brain," center for emotionality) are theorized to take precedence over higher centers in the neocortex (especially the prefrontal lobes), producing *animal cunning and obsessive-compulsive, ritualistic behavior.*

Animal cunning trumps human intelligence (reason) most of the time. Why? Because cunning is fast-talking and deliberate, almost knee-jerk action: psychopaths are able to dodge detection through duplicity—the familiar smoke and mirrors. That's why it takes thirty years in some cases to catch these birds in rapacious activity—defined as *preying upon others.* In more ways than most of us care to know it really is a jungle out there. In the age of "cool-coded" brain scans showing reduced capacity of frontal lobes—the "brakes" of psychosocial behavior—it's time to wake up and smell the coffee.

The "social" psychopath may be a president, a religious leader, or a national sports hero. He may even live next door. Regardless, he is a sexual magnet to many young women who should know better. But, the seduction is in full swing almost immediately with a smile that could "melt" rock hard candy. Sexual innuendo is part of the charm. He's exciting to be around. He has such a great sense of humor. He's a risk taker. What lies beneath? The answer is a master manipulator and con artist. When females finally get their fill of his prevarication and parasitic lifestyle, they're ready to move on and find a guy suitable to take home and meet the parents. In the meantime, she may actually give him one or two more chances. In which case, girlfriends (as well as others with "dealings") continue to be seduced by his convincing persona. Is Charles Manson in the house?

Social psychopaths seek stimulation because they bore easily. (Most have been diagnosed as ADD or ADHD by age ten and were not good students although some were Rhodes Scholars.) As adolescents and young adults (under thirty years of age) they are extraverts—people, parties, and darkness stimulated them as "night crawlers" seeking "prey." They take plenty from girlfriends and others (with whom they have "dealings") and give practically nothing back—except more of themselves, which they are certain they have plenty to spare. They routinely disappoint those who feel close to them and have "stood by their man." They are in and out of many "intimate" relationships. They're over their last relationship before it's over. Pay attention those of you in Yogi Berra's Learning Center—with psychopaths it's over before it's over!

The severe psychopath is the worst kind of criminal. He is a sexual predator. The world knows him as a serial killer. In his twenties to mid-thirties, the sexual psychopath develops by virtue of five influences: hateful, antisocial parenting (the worst kind of loveless parenting imaginable), deviant cognitive mapping (sexually perverted thinking),

(continues)

(continued)

irreverible neurological brain damage (showing "cool-coded" brain scans), addiction to hardcore, violent pornography, and poly-addiction (such as alcoholism and/or substance abuse, and addiction to his own twisted brain chemistry). There is no treatment for sexual psychopathy. Lock them up and throw away the key. Or, euthanize them and don't take ten years. *Milder versions of psychopaths just wreck lives and cause emotional havoc with whom they have had "dealings."*

Darwin spoke of survival of the fittest through natural selection. Milder psychopathy may be why some survive the jungle and others fail. Caring for others and their welfare takes valuable time and energy away fromt he cognitive focus required in rapacious behavior. Psychopaths are willing to spill a little blood and sweat but never tears, unless the tears are of the crocodile version.

Narcissism and histrionic behavior demand a lot of attention and adoration so it's only natural that psychopaths make terrific leaders. Seldom do others see what lies beneath the surface and how pervasive psychopathy really is. In a case of speculative irony, perhaps the mark of the beast in Revelations 13: 16–18 is the *psychopathic "killer"* (literally or figuratively). It does add up: *Psycho + pathic + killer*—six letters each or 666. Interesting.

Run by a small lithium battery charged by changes in skin temperature, a microchip courtesy of *quantum mechanics* is forthcoming as a kind of "electric" Prozac engineered to control damaged brain centers through electrical stimulation. Almost two million dollars later, researchers discovered the parts of the skin most sensitive to temperture changes are the forehead and hand. Take another look at verse sixteen.

A major glitch for psychopaths is elementary: they never learn. They are guided by routine and ritualistic behavior and the worst kind of arrogant egoism. This strange brew of chemical-driven behavior passes for confidence for those not skilled in identifying what lies beneath. Attention shoppers!—if he seems to good to be true, he is too good to be true. Period. A little psychopathy goes a long way. A mature psychopath (over forty years of age) with moderate psychopathy and a dose of egoism may go undetected or many years, unless "bizarre" circumstances unmask him. But, his psychopathic character has always been there just below the surface. From childhood, his cunning has been growing, developing, and strangely nurturing. For mild, moderate, and severe psychopaths, the train wreck is going to happen, it's just a matter of when. (It took years for Ohio State's Woody Hays to finally strike a player.) Anger is a big part of psychopathy festering just below surface shine. The only ingredient missing is the "triggering" event, and it might just be "bizarre."—Don Jacobs, 2003

■ Eight Psychological Perspectives— Underlying the Study of Sexual Psychopathy

The following **psychological perspectives** are known to underlie the analysis and identification of **psychopathy** (analyzing, describing, and diagnosing psychopathic personality). Tangentially, they constitute the underpinnings of the "mousetrap"—the criminal profile—so effective in targeting serial predators. (In our nomenclature the term "serial predator" means *serial killer,* or *sexual psychopath.* The following principles will be identified, defined, and analyzed throughout subsequent chapters as perspectives important in profiling psychopathy.

Behavioral Psychology Perspective

(1) Behavioral psychology (**behaviorism**) focuses on learned behavioral *patterns and habits* in various social **milieus** (social contexts of learning) as formative influences in the developmental programming of psychopathy (as well as normal behavior). FBI profilers contend "behavior lies behind personality," hence a knowledge of *behavioral psychology* is essential in connecting the "dots" of behavior—habits and patterns—of psychopathic personality. **Antisocial parenting,** highlighted by severe physical and/or sexual abuse that emotionally and physically "disfigures" childhood and adolescent behavior, leaves "red flags" behind such as **enuresis** (at an inappropriate age), cruelties to animals and peers, and fire-setting. Most notably, both physical abuse and emotional abuse produces *irreversible neurological brain damage* in the brains of "becoming" psychopaths. Startling neurological brain imaging presented in Chapter Five documents "**cool-coded**" prefrontal lobe damage (as well as to other brain areas such as the temporal lobes and cerebellum) from sophisticated brain scanning technology.

Parenthetically, the general term *behaviorism* refers to the distinctly North American perspective in psychology rooted in *direct observation, cause and effect,* and **empiricism**—laboratory proof, analysis, and reporting. Behavioral psychology seeks *empirical verification* exemplified by the rigorous laboratory forensic evidence extracted from crime scenes by **forensic pathologists.**

Today, criminal investigation and criminal prosecution are 99% *driven by forensic evidence,* except for one notable exception. Which one? Unscramble the following letters to find out: snoojmpsi seca* (when you give up, see the bottom of the next page).

It is no wonder that the behavioristic approach to understand violent, criminal behavior is favored over the more speculative **intrapsychic** hunches (speculation based on "self-reports") observed in various *psychodynamic* perspectives focusing on unconscious motivation a lá Dr. Freud.

Interestingly, Ressler and other FBI agents obtained similar "self-reports" from incarcerated serial perpetrators encouraged to talk about aspects of their crimes. Somewhat **cathartic**, the perpetrators got a chance to gloat one more time about their crimes. In the process, agents benefited by learning more about "what makes them tick." The *self-report* accounts for almost 100% of *known offender characteristics* based on direct face-to-face interviews with incarcerated offenders. Contrary to strict behavioral psychology, self-reports from incarcerated criminals have proven to be quite accurate, and have been indispensable in the development of criminal profiling.

The specialty field of (2) **forensic psychology** is characterized by testimony from **forensic psychologists and neuropsychologists**—psychologists who specialize in criminal behavior and the startling new evidence from brains scans that have created so much debate in the courtroom.

These highly paid professionals provide expert insight into crime scene evidence, brain scans, and the state of mind of the perpetrator, as well as strategies in insanity pleas. With neuroscience firmly planted in the courtroom, first-degree murder can be mitigated to second-degree murder (hence a sentence of life in prison instead of a death sentence) due to such compelling "proof" from "cool-coded" brain scans. Forensic psychology has deep roots in both criminology and behavioral psychology. **Forensic neuropsychology** has deep roots in biology, neurology, and medicine.

Cognitive-Behavioral Perspective

The (3) **cognitive-behavioral** perspective of psychology, otherwise known as "soft" behaviorism, focuses on the relationship between *aberrant thinking, focus, and motivation* producing powerful "cognitive maps" of behavior. (In the case of sexual psychopathy, deviant and perverted "maps" of erotic fantasies are theorized to produce **rapacious** crime—crimes of rape and murder—by sexual psychopaths preying upon unsuspecting victims. This perspective, more than any other principle, explains why an *addiction to hardcore violent pornography* upon a neurologically damaged brain is central to the expression of sexualized violence. Connecting the two perspectives—cognitive (thinking) and behavioral (acting) is a perfect metaphor for the interconnectedness of mind-body, the current model of **holism** in behavioral neuroscience.

Abnormal Psychology Perspective

Abnormal psychology, or (4) **psychopathology**, targets dysfunctional family relationships, pure psychopathologies (such as paranoid schizophrenia, bipolar affective disorder, and **DID** (dissociative identity disorder). In serial crime, the perspective documents severe **personality disorder**, such as **antisocial personality**. Often, a history of precursor "red flags" in childhood and adolescence (such as **Conduct Disorder** or **Oppositional Defiant Disorder**) is observed. Discussed at length in upcoming chapters, features of antisocial, narcissistic, and borderline personality disorders may also exacerbate sexual psychopathy.

---

*O.J. Simpson case

Developmental Psychology Perspective

(5) **Developmental psychology** in the tradition of Erik Erikson's classic *psychosocial stages* of "lifespan" development, targets unsatisfied emotional "crises" brought about by incompetent parenting, not to mention hateful, antisocial parenting. Primate studies of **tactile stimulation**, (i.e. Harlow and Bowlby) which produces emotional scarcity, lack of attachment, and lack of bonding is known to *retard* brain development.

Severe neurological deficits in cerebellar development, the brain area most affected by lack of tactile and motor stimulation (in most instances before age 2), pathologically "rewires" neurological systems making conventional "talk therapy" completely ineffective as a treatment protocol.

■ Neuropsychology & Addictionology

"Compelled" versus "Choice" Behavior

The compatible disciplines of (6) **neuropsychology** and (7) **addictionology** identifies powerful neurotransmitters and neurohormones underlying normal thinking and behavior and how the identical chemistry becomes *perverted* in psychopathy due to addiction and the developmental insults of physical, sexual, and verbally abusive antisocial parenting. Understanding addiction and its effect on neurological systems provides insight into *compelled* behavior versus so-called *choice* behavior due to the devastation of neurological systems. Severe neurological abnormalities in *cognitive mapping* are exacerbated with addiction to hardcore violent pornography, documented by authorities as the single most devastating influence in adult sexualized crimes.

■ Evolutionary Neuroanatomy

(8) **Evolutionary neuroanatomy** of brain development according to neurologist Paul McLean's **reptilian brain theory** can no longer be ignored as part of the irreversible demonic "cocktail of psychopathy" in neurochemistry and hormones of sexual psychopaths.

■ Criminal Profiling—Three Important Terms in Sexual Psychopathy: "Serial," "MO," and "Signature"

Serial

Former Special Agent to the FBI, Robert Ressler (*Whoever Fights Monsters*) is given credit for coining the term "serial killers." Ressler chose the term "serial" after hearing a speaker at the British police academy refer to "crimes in a series"—a series of crimes attributed to the same offender. Shown before the feature attraction in movie theaters, the word conjured up in Ressler's mind the series of short films he enjoyed as a kid. The short reel "serials" presented sequential segments as a marketing tool to entice moviegoers to come back each Saturday and watch the next installment. Cowboys and Indians, *Buck Rogers,* and the *Adventures of Zorro* were popular serials.

Word usage from one venue can be used effectively in another so that everyday activities can be observed using the "serial" moniker and the well-known evidentiary tools of criminal law—*modus operandi* and signature. For example, a textbook author writing a series of books can be referred to as a *serial author.* One book follows another with a "cooling off" period between publications. The "cooling off" period refers to any breaks the author takes from writing, such as doing basic research on another book, or simply taking a mental break from writing altogether.

MO: *Modus Operandi*

Legal scholars use the term *modus operandi*—the procedure or method of operation used by a given criminal at the crime scene, reflecting "how he did it." In authoring a college text, what comprises *MO?* The book you hold in your hands provides an example. Jacobs' first effort at producing a college text occurred in 1996 after being displeased with standard adoptions. Jacobs bundled together a collection of pop culture articles relating to the course material (the course was Intro Psych) as "enhancement readings" to accompany the text. Immediately, students indicated they found the articles more enjoyable and informative and preferred the handouts to the text.

Jacobs discovered that most Introductory Psychology texts are too long and too impersonal for use in pedagogy he believes should focus on group interaction in the classroom. Also, many standard texts fall far short of providing enough quality information related to pop culture, an extremely important social milieu for college students. As the years went by, he expanded the pop culture materials and wrote introductory material suitable for group interaction and discussion. Applied psychology became the focus of his texts. At this point, the articles were rewritten in the author's own conversational style focusing on expanding *scholarly lexica*—word knowledge.

In all, the author's first "text" contained approximately 300 pages "shrink wrapped" in cellophane, unstapled, hand numbered at the bottom of the pages, and sold in the college bookstore. Soon, a publisher showed interest and custom published the work.

Subsequent texts *evolved* from Jacobs' original *MO*—pop culture articles mixed with standard textbook material, including shorter, more conversational-style paragraphs, more application exercises, and the *ever-present focus* on learning *scholarly vocabulary*—the *Word Scholar* component. Jacobs' *MO* continued to evolve and change, aided by more student involvement (at one time, pictures of outstanding students were featured on the cover and throughout the text).

Slowly, through experience, the author became a more experienced writer, more descriptive of pop culture insights, and more convinced that student contributions were critical to producing an effective text. The title of the introductory text evolved from all of the aforementioned as *Psychology: Brain, Behavior, and Popular Culture,* now in its fourth edition.

Just like serial crimes, the *modus operandi* of textbook writing—how the text developed from inception through continual evolution—is always dynamic, always changeable, and always based upon feedback and experiences of what "works" and what "doesn't work", just like the *MO* of criminal behavior.

Signature: *Cri de Coeur*

What comprises the *signature* of a sexually inspired crime? In crime scene analysis, signature represents a given serial predator's *emotionally compelling reason* why he committed the crime in the first place. *What emotionally fulfills* him by the *nature of his crime* defines signature.

Based upon an analysis of this text and other texts by the same author, what constitutes Jacobs' textbook signature? Discovering the *one indispensable motivation* running through his textbooks discloses signature.

The one unchanging ingredient in all of the Jacobs texts is his passion for *word knowledge* represented as *Word Scholar.* The focus on scholarly words and word knowledge helps compose powerful *cognitive maps of experience,* almost single-handedly forging the *scholarly mindset,* which is the author's signature. Appropriately, this philosophical persuasion embraces the expanding field of **neuropsycholinguists**—how language knowledge functions to enrich the human experience and *enhance personality* by feeling "scholarly." Jacobs' focus on scholarly words is not necessary to writing the text, but it is the reason—the *cri de coeur*—the "passionate cry from the heart" for doing so.

Readers, take a moment to analyze the following *psychosocial activities* in relation to serialization, *MO,* and signature.

1. Dating behavior is serial behavior. You go out, come home, do something else—comprising "cooling off" period. What is your MO? What is your *method of operation* (always tied to feedback) on dates? What is your signature dating behavior—what emotionally jazzes you so that your dating partner can expect it on each date?
2. Sexual behavior is serial behavior. Describe a possible MO scenario from one partner to another. Define a possible signature?
3. What is MO and signature for "breakup behavior," or "jealousy behavior"?

■ The Meat of the Matter—Profundity of Psychopathy

Criminal profiling is most useful to investigators when the crime scene reflects a more *profound degree of psychopathology* as observed at the crime scene. According to Holmes & Holmes, and verified by FBI statistics, criminal profiling offers the *best chance of targeting the probable offender* relative to the following crimes:

1. Sadistic torture/sadistic assaults
2. **Evisceration**
3. **Postmortem** slashing/cutting
4. **Pyromania**
5. Lust/mutilation murders
6. Rape
7. Satanic/ritualistic crimes
8. **Pedophilia**

The justification for the **efficacy** of profiling the aforementioned select group of crimes will be addressed in forthcoming chapters. For the time being, the guiding principle of profiling predators who commit *sexually driven crimes* requires perpetrators to have (1) a depraved mind, and (2) severely flawed character defined by (3) lack of restraint, and (4) emotional apathy toward victims. In a nutshell, this describes the *psychopathic personality with sexual psychopathy*.

Due to the heinous nature of serial crimes and the societal unrest engendered by serial rapes and murders, human predators are dangerous every second of freedom they have due to the rapacious crimes they commit.

■ The Whitechapel Murderer— "Jack the Ripper"

Jack the Ripper is the first subject of *Predator Profiles*—selected bios of serial killers—strategically placed in intervening chapters (except Chapter Eight). The Ripper is interesting for a number of reasons. First, his identity is still unknown and will probably never be known. Therefore, Jack the Ripper is an **UNSUB** (*unidentified subject* in FBI lingo).

In 1888, the term "serial killer" did not exist. As we have seen, it would take over 90 years before criminal profiling was introduced to public scrutiny in the Atlanta child murders.

Second, The Ripper killed prostitutes. He mutilated corpses. He displayed a *modus operandi* and signature. Hollywood presented films on the Ripper, a 1970s installment with the unlikely choice of matinee idol Tony Curtis as the Ripper. Recently, *From Hell,* starring Johnny Depp as a clairvoyant criminal investigator, pricked our collective unconsciousness but raised more questions than answers. Today, we might know the identity of Jack the Ripper if only an experienced agent could use time travel to survey the crime scenes.

PREDATOR PROFILE (1-1)

UNSUB
"Jack the Ripper"

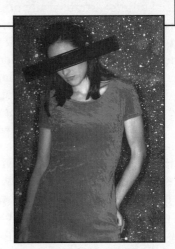

Alternative Media Monikers:

Saucy Jack
Whitechapel Murderer
Autumn of Terror

Time Span Crimes Committed:

August 31, 1888—November 9, 1888

Physical Description of Offender:

Unknown

Offenses Prior to Serial Killing:

Unknown

MO & Victimology:

Compliant prostitutes were killed and then "ripped" open. Each crime occurred in an isolated area (all but the last was outdoors); each crime scene provided means of easy escape. The Ripper and his victims stood facing each other. Victims were distracted by voluntarily lifting their skirts. The Ripper strangled the victims until unconscious or dead.

Signature:

Victims were lowered to the ground after strangling and positioned with their head tilted to the victim's right side. Victims' throats were slashed with straight razor blade (from left to right) with victim positioned as above (evidence of blood splatter at scene indicates most of the victims were dead by strangulation prior to having the throat cut). Violent post-mortem mutilation, usually including graphic positioning of eviscerated intestines suggested hatred for women or the profession of prostitution.

Collection of trophies varied, but included: visceral tissue, kidney, uterus, heart or ears. Bodies were left at the crime scene. There was no apparent ante-mortem or post-mortem sexual activity with the victim.

Current Status:

Unsolved and apparently will remain unsolved forever.

Comments:

Due to signature, the murderer had some knowledge of anatomy and physiology. Some letters received by newspapers contained information that only the killer could have known. During the time the killer was most active, police organized frequent sweeps of the East End. The Ripper may have been among the persons incarcerated for other crimes, or he may have been sent to an insane asylum.

Police "sweeps" may have taken Jack the Ripper off the streets permanently, accounting for the sudden cessation of the serial killings.

Organized versus Disorganized:

The Ripper crimes have elements consistent with the *disorganized* type of killer. The similarity and proximity of locations indicate a person not traveling far from his residence, and the violence of the post-mortem mutilation. At the same time, The Ripper had enough cognizance (awareness) and social skills to consistently identify and solicit the same type of victims (prostitutes), to vary his MO (the last victim was killed indoors and was also the most brutally eviscerated), and to perform the same ritualistic methods (throat slashing, followed by post-mortem mutilation). If the killer were the person who wrote some of the taunting letters to the newspapers, this fact would point toward a more **hedonistic** personality, and therefore, a more *organized* killer.

Names of Victims:

Mary Ann Nichols
Annie Chapman
Elizabeth Stride
Catherine Eddowes
Mary Jane Kelly (a movie, *Mary Kelly* starring Julia Roberts depicted her life with fictional and non-fictional aspects)

Names of Possible Suspects:

Francis Thompson (poet, drug user, failed medical student).
John Pizer (butcher, ruled out as suspect by police).
Michael Ostrogg (Russian, physician, known to use aliases).
Alexander Pedachenko (Russian, physician, possibly the same person as Michael Ostrogg, who returned to Russia and eventually died in mental asylum).
Aaron Kisminski (Jewish, Polish immigrant, began time in insane asylums in 1890, probably schizophrenic).
HRH Prince Albert Victor—The Duke of Clarence (pure speculation).

Student Contributors:

Jacki Arwood, Faie LaFleur, Clarissa Noland, Nia Nolen, Brettne Sanders, PA and Rae Ellen Wooten, PA

ALTERNATIVE COMMENTARY: *"The Ripper"*

Mary Ann Nichols, Annie Chapman, Elizabeth Stride, Catherine Eddowes, and Mary Jane Kelly were prostitutes in the seedy suburb of Whitechapel in the final days of Victorian London. Contrary to the movies, none of the ladies knew each other; in fact, none of the ladies had any particular striking similarities but one on the last night of their lives; they each lifted their skirts to the same killer.

For over a century, speculation abounds regarding the identity of the killer. With his MO and signature of postmortem slashing of the victims' throats, and retrieval of a fleshly trophy, it was presumed the killer had some intimate knowledge of human anatomy. Was the Ripper an anonymous midwife who abhorred the morally perverse lifestyle of the prostitutes? Could it have been Montague John Druitt, an incompetent attorney whose suicide coincided with the cessation of the killer's activities? Perhaps Dr. Roslyn D'Onston Stephenson, an author and magician, performed the killings as part of a dark satanic ritual of empowerment. And, of course, the most salacious speculation centered on HRH Prince Albert Victor, Duke of Clarence and grandson to Queen Victoria. Occasionally, even police officers and constables were suspected.

Despite recent investigations and incisive analysis by such crime writers as crime-novelist Patricia Cornwell and FBI profiler, turned true crime author Robert Ressler, there remains as much mystery today regarding the identity of the Ripper as was evident in the late fall of 1888. Were letters to the newspapers purportedly written by the killer authentic or an ignominious fabrication? What caused the killer to suddenly stop? Was he incarcerated for another crime, or perhaps incarcerated in an insane asylum?

The greatest of all crime mysteries—Who was Jack the Ripper?—will forever remain unsolved. It has been over a hundred years since Jack the Ripper killed his last victim. The dead may "chatter" to forensic specialists, but the name was never uttered to anyone who lived to tell.

Student Contributor:

Rae Ellen Wooten, PA

Alternative Theory:

Sir Arthur Canon Doyle speculated a man dressed as a woman was "Jack the Ripper." Offer evidence to support this view.

■ Applied Forensic Criminology—Known Offender Characteristics

By merging principles of psychology with forensic science and *known offender characteristics* in computerized databases, present and future cases have a criminal "yardstick" for reference. Therefore, the method of capturing serial predators is termed **inductive**, rather than deductive. In this way, systematized knowledge replaces speculation or "hunches" (used by the famous fictional detective Sherlock Holmes), edging profiling ever closer to science. However, experienced profilers contend profiling is also "artwork"—it depends on speculative logic, common sense, and sometimes, sheer luck. Non-scientific "yardsticks" of reference produce philosophical speculation known as **deductive reasoning**. In the words of ex-FBI profiler John Douglas, "the more you know about a predator's 'artwork' the more you know about the 'artist.'"

FBI computers at the *National Center for the Analysis of Violent Crimes (NCAVC)* are filled with the nightmarish accounts of dysfunctional histories, sexual obsessions, and macabre fascination, all of which comprise the *behavioral dynamics* of society's most elusive predators. From this growing database, profilers, relying on the principles of behavioral science, peer inside the mind of serial rapists and killers to see what "makes them tick".

Hence, forensic science depends on *systematized knowledge* (the organized information and methodology of behavioral science) applied by forensic psychologists and forensic psychiatrists as well as other criminal investigators in studying serial predators. (The word *forensic* means information "headed to the courtroom"), hence a **forensic pathologist** investigates physical evidence at the crime scene, such as wound patterns, ligature (strangulation) marks, specific physical trauma to the victim, DNA traces, and related evidence used in court.

In contrast, a **forensic psychologist** might be asked to testify in court regarding *behavioral characteristics* of the offender suggested by the crime scene, or the feasibility of an insanity plea. Both the pathologist (MD-credentialed, such as celebrated pathologists Dr. Henry Lee and Dr. Michael Baden) and the psychologist (PhD- credentialed) lend their expertise to courtroom proceedings.

Currently, the FBI is the largest investigative group engaged in violent crime profiling; however, retired special agents of the FBI (such as John Douglas, the first full-time profiler at the FBI's *Behavioral Science Unit* and Robert Ressler, co-founder of the modern system of profiling) offer expertise as private consultants.

However, since the terrorism of 9/11, the FBI has been "retooled" in some respects to investigate *only the most publicized violent crimes*. Terrorism is now the main focus of the FBI's latest attempt to redefine itself in light of the current homeland *zeitgeist*. As important as abolishing terrorism is, what will become of less publicized serial crimes on the already overburdened metropolitan police forces? We shudder to think.

■ Multiple Murder Defined

Criminologists delineate three types of multiple murder categories. A **serial killer**, the focus of this text, murders at least three victims followed by an emotional "cooling off" period between crimes. Ted Bundy, Jeffrey Dahmer, and the fictional "Buffalo Bill", from the Thomas Harris novel *Silence of the Lambs,* qualify as serial killers. (A serial rapist, of course, rapes sequentially.)

A **mass murderer** murders four or more victims in one location in one incident and in one emotional experience. From his perch high atop the Texas Tower at the University of Texas, Austin, sniper Charles Whitman killed twelve students at random in the early 1960s. Along with Whitman, Richard Speck, who killed eight nursing students on a Chicago college campus, fits the definition of mass murderers. A **spree killer** is defined as a rampaging perpetrator who murders in at least two or more locations with no emotional "cooling off" period.

The FBI describes serial killers as the most *cunning and sinister of all violent criminals.* Monetary gain is not the motivator, nor is a "heat of passion" murder observed in involuntary manslaughter. *Preying upon others for perverted sexual gratification is the driving force behind serial crime.* As we previously noted, this delineates the *sexual psychopath* from all other varieties of psychopathic personalities.

Almost impossible to capture or to predict his next move using ordinary investigative methods, serial predators are ironically (and perversely) attracted to the police who pursue them. Many are police "buffs" who impersonate police officers as a **ruse** to gain quicker access to targeted victims. Some serial criminals attend news conferences related to the crimes they have committed or routinely visit cemeteries where their victims are buried.

■ Aspects of Serial Homicide

Serial homicides are almost always *intraracial;* that is, white offenders kill white victims, black offenders kill black victims and so on. However, for reasons largely unknown, most offenders are almost always white males, twenty to mid-thirty years of age. In the initial stages of a suspected serial homicide, FBI profilers begin with age 25 for the *UNSUB* and then add or subtract years based on *sophistication* of the crime scene.

Clearly, years of interviewing serial murderers by authorities show that no individual, regardless of ethnicity or race, simply wakes up one morning (at any age) and decides to kill a string of strangers.

It is well known that becoming a serial predator starts with years of *systematic abuse* in severely dysfunctional families characterized by antisocial parenting. Societal "safety nets"—schools and churches—failed them as much as destructive parenting. In dysfunctional milieus, *pathological personality* develops in young adolescent males headed into serial crime. (Chapter Seven analyzes the dysfunctional influences in family milieu in the development of adolescent "Rambo" killers.)

Due to extensive neurological brain damage, serial killers have little respect for self or others; pre-adolescent and adolescents who are "becoming" serial killers feel little or no remorse or guilt for killing animals, stealing, hurting other children or pets, or setting fires—some of the more recognizable "red flags" of psychopathy. (We use the term "becoming" throughout the text to denote the slowly "simmering," soon-to-emerge serial predator as a function of *antecedent* dysfunctional experiences, developmental glitches, and/or inadequate neurological inactivity in select brain areas).

Inner "demons" of rage torment the future killer as the tentacles of dysfunction squeeze away any hope of normalcy in the life of the future rapist/murderer. The anger at being "different" eats away at fragile self-esteem. As experienced profilers know, it doesn't happen any other way.

Serial predators operate just "below the radar" of law enforcement and beyond the relentless pursuit of authorities. Some move from state to state, retreating into the background on occasion, only to emerge again in different geographical parts of the country to continue more of the *seemingly motiveless killings*. Yet, serial homicide *always has a motive*. Serial killers are obsessed with keeping the victim alive as long as possible since *serial predators sexualize every aspect of killing from fantasy to aftermath.* They seek control, domination, degradation; they seek sexual experimentation, sometimes observed as torture and humiliation. The desire to repeat the sexualized crimes operates as an obsession, swiftly becoming a compulsion, leading to full-blown addiction to rapacious crime.

■ Personality Disorder NOS and Dual Diagnosis

In the *DSM (Diagnostic and Statistical Manual of Mental Disorders)* terminology, a convincing argument exists that most serial killers should be diagnosed with **personality disorder** NOS (not otherwise specified) due to the presence of *two or more personality disorders*. The characteristic antisocial personality (e.g. the **colloquial** "psychopathic personality"), while satisfying the general classification of antisocial behavior, misses features of **narcissism** and/or **histrionic personality disorder** (covered in a later chapter).

Perhaps more importantly, serial predators present a **dual diagnosis**; that is, they display one or more personality disorders as well as *two or more chemical addictions,* such as pornography, sex, alcoholism, or other chemical dependencies. The complexity of numerous personality disorders and addictions upon cognition and emotion explains why *no single root cause* of sexual psychopathy will ever be identified, nor should be.

Addicted to the "thrilling high" of raping or killing another human as if it were a drug, serial predators compulsively seek victims in the following targeted areas:

1. Shopping malls, parks, and school playgrounds,
2. City streets under cover of darkness,

3. Country roads in isolated rural communities,
4. In broad daylight in congested areas, or
5. Anyplace, USA where victims are perceived to be vulnerable (as inattentive adults "chaperoning" children in a crowded mall).

Like wolves who survey large herds of animals for the next meal by seeking out the weak, the elderly, the sickly, or the inattentive—any member who slows the herd down—similarly, serial predators seek out *personal characteristics* of naïve victims that "turn him on" sexually. For example, Ted Bundy favored young girls with long brown hair, split down the middle. Every serial rapist/murder has his favorite physical type.

Increasingly, across North America it is sobering that common areas of high statistical probability for serial crimes are apartment complexes, college campuses, nightclubs, and darkened streets where prostitutes work. Routinely, serial predators cruise lonely country roads as well as busy metropolitan streets trolling for victims. Being at the wrong place at the right time can have devastating consequences. Hovering around convenience stores is becoming a favorite spot to snatch unattended children. Citizens should be able to move at will through society without fear of being a statistic of serial crime. However, it is becoming painfully obvious that citizens—especially women, children, and parents of children—must be aware of the potential dangers of serial predators. Never has the idiom "an ounce of prevention is worth a pound of cure" been more applicable.

No longer are any neighborhoods 100% safe.

It is good advice for families to watch children like hawks because someone else may swoop down and steal them right out of front yards. Therefore, the *cri de coeur*—the passionate cry from the heart underlying the presentation of this material—is *consciousness raising*. Predators exist and move freely through society. Citizens and law enforcers must embrace ways of recognition, protection, and apprehension of the monsters that hide behind human faces.

◼ Whoever Fights Monsters

The behavior of both the hunter (profiler) and the hunted (perpetrator) are subject to the tools of behavioral psychology. With so many instances of dysfunction, profilers are alerted to the dangers of "getting inside the head" of predators, as Robert Ressler states in his book *Whoever Fights Monsters* (quoting Friedrich Nietzsche)

> ". . . Whoever fights monsters should see to it that in the process he does not become a monster. And when you look into the abyss (the depraved mind of the serial killer), the abyss also looks into you."

John Douglas recounts his mental and emotional meltdown as a consequence of becoming "too absorbed" with serial criminals in his book *Journey Into Darkness* (1997).

"Those who study serial predators are not alarmists seeking to scare the wits out of readers. Instead, we seek to educate and inform others of the dangers of serial killers whose ghastly acts taunt authorities with "catch me if you can" mentality. Control is a focal point of serial predators (of the organized variety), who decide when and where to strike. Upon apprehension, serial predators perceive being caught as mere luck; they remain arrogant, believing they are still smarter than the police."

■ The "Trigger" & Compulsion of Serial Offenses

To serial killers, the first murder leaves them in an emotional "no exit" situation. The killer is left feeling perhaps ambivalent. On the one hand, the "thrilling high" of finally actualizing fantasy is mixed with the cold irreversible reality of being a killer. In his mind, there is no exit. Once the line is crossed from fantasy to murder, he will be forever a criminal. Whether or not his psyche is tortured, he has killed another human. How does he draw back from that and live a normal life?

Holding back the urge to kill someone sooner or later must be addressed. Often, the presence of a precipitation "trigger" leads to an escalation of murderous impulses. The two most common psychological "triggers" are (1) loss of work (income), and (2) loss of a love interest. The flimsy "dam" of restraint unleashes a tidal wave of sexualized fantasies, rage, and ultimately *emotional non-fulfillment,* according to Robert Ressler, former special agent of the FBI.

■ Serial Killer or Wrong Man Convicted?

Could outcry from the public be so intense in finding serial perpetrators that the wrong person is convicted? Take the case of William Heirens. Seventeen-year-old Bill Heirens was a petty thief. Near one of his burglaries, a female victim of murder was discovered. A vicious attack upon a child whose torso washed up in a drain sewer suggested a serial killer was on the prowl. The press was frantic to find the killer. Was Bill in the wrong place at the right time? Did police "torture" the young petty burglar into confession to save him from the death penalty? Was Heirens the "Lipstick Killer"?

PREDATOR PROFILE (1-2)

William Heirens
"The Lipstick Killer"

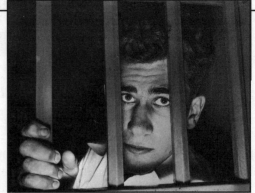

©Bettmann/CORBIS

A Serial Killer or Wrong Man Convicted?

Personal Background

William George Heirens (HY-renz) was born November 15, 1928 to George and Margaret Heirens. Heirens and his younger brother Jere were raised in Chicago, Illinois, where their father worked at various odd jobs around the time of World War II. Due to financial difficulties, both children stayed with babysitters while their mother was forced to work to help balance the family budget. Heirens' father often escaped his family obligations by drinking and spending time with friends, which led to frequent arguments at home.

With his own method of coping with the situation at home, Heirens began a life of petty crime at an early age (criminal "priors" are common in serial killers). After his first arrest at the age of 13 for carrying a loaded gun in connection with petty burglaries, Heirens was sent to the Catholic Gibault School for troubled youths in Terre Haute, Indiana. Later, Heirens was sent to the St. Bede's Academy following additional charges of burglary.

Despite his early life of crime and problems at home, Heirens was an excellent student (not common among serial killers). With an estimated I.Q. of 129, he was accepted into The University of Chicago at the age of 16. In college, Heirens was an intelligent, handsome young man, and had no apparent difficulties in making friends. Despite his academic success, lacking money necessary to maintain his social activities, Heirens continued the pattern of burglary.

Overview of Murders

On June 5, 1945, Josephine Ross was found murdered at her Chicago apartment. The victim was stabbed several times in the throat with a knife. Despite the fact that the apartment was in total disarray, police investigators found no fingerprints at the scene. The victim's stab wounds had been bandaged after her body had been washed in the sink by the perpetrator. Only a small amount of change was found to be missing from the victim's apartment.

On December 10, 1945, Francine Brown, an honorably discharged US Navy WAVE, was found murdered in her Chicago apartment. She died from two stab wounds to the neck and two bullet wounds in the head. Similar to the previous victim, the perpetrator had washed her body in the bathtub after the crime, apparently. Again, police investigators found the room in total disarray but nothing of any value was missing. On the wall in the victim's apartment were the words, *"For heaven's sake, catch me before I kill more. I cannot control myself."*

Less than one month later, Suzanne Degnan, a six-year-old girl, was taken from her bed in the middle of the night. She was taken to the basement of an empty laundry, where she was strangled and her body chopped into pieces. Various parts of her body would later be discovered in the sewers located throughout Chicago. While the public was alarmed after the first two murders, the circumstances surrounding the murder of Suzanne Degnan pushed the public into panic. Police investigators came under increasing pressure from both the citizens of Chicago as well as the local news media to solve all three seemingly related crimes.

Soon after, police investigators reported a major breakthrough in the ongoing investigation, when seventeen-year-old William Heirens was apprehended during a failed burglary attempt. Heirens had been caught in the act by two off-duty police officers. A struggle ensued, in which Heirens drew a gun on the officers. The gun misfired and Heirens was apprehended and brought in for questioning. Police officials strongly believed that the man apprehended was the killer for whom they had been searching. From this point on it was a media circus until Heirens, near exhaustion from police questioning, finally confessed. In all there were 157 headline stories about the case before he finally confessed to the murders.

Physical Description

17-year-old handsome white male
University of Chicago student
IQ of 129
Dark brown hair
Slender build

Span of time Crimes Committed

During the years 1941–1946

Media Moniker

At first, the media referred to Heirens as "Murder Man," stemming from his alter ego George Murman, which Heirens referred to during police interrogation under the influence of Sodium Pentothal. (Profiler Robert Ressler postulated "Murman" meant "murder man.") This label was later changed to the notorious "Lipstick Killer," taken from the message left at the apartment of Francine Brown.

Victimology

The killer changed his MO from murdering two adult females to kidnapping and killing a six-year-old child. No money or other items of value were taken from any of the crime scenes, with the exception of the pocket change taken from the apartment of Josephine Ross. Although a ransom note was found at the scene of Suzanne Degnan's murder, no reasonable attempt was made to follow through on the demands. The only apparent motives were control and domination over the victims' fate.

Heirens left the famous lipstick message on the wall: "For heaven's sake, catch me before I kill more. I cannot control myself." Additionally, he also left a ransom note in Suzanne Degan's room in his own words which read: "Get $20,000 Ready + Waite for Word. Do Not Notify FBI or Police. Bills in 5's and 10's. BURN THIS FOR HER SAFETY."

Psychological Issues

Heirens fit the pattern of *antisocial personality disorder* (psychopathic personality) to the extent (1) he was unable to learn from his mistakes (2) he had a proven pattern of stealing, lying, and delinquency, and (3) he complained of tension, depression and boredom (a need for frequent stimulation).

In the course of the police interrogation, Heirens mentioned his alter ego he referred to as "George Murman." The police deduced Heirens was faking, although doctors initially believed that he showed signs of schizophrenia. Heirens later recanted the alter ego story. Also, Heirens admitted suffering from sexual problems and deficient coping skills due to family dysfunction and lack of communication.

According to Journalist Lucy Freeman in her book, *Before I Kill More*:

"To explain the method in Bill's killings, two things must be considered—what psychiatrists call 'the predisposition toward' the deed and the 'precipitating factor' . . . If (his) foundation of life is one of *excessive fear and anger* which pervades (his) whole life, then (he) is said to have a 'predisposition toward' murder. The 'precipitating factor' is the straw that broke Bill's 'psychic back,' allowing the anger to erupt into violence."

Current Status

At age of seventy-five, Heirens is serving three consecutive life sentences awarded him by the state of Illinois. Now a diabetic, he suffers from numerous health problems. Both of his parents are deceased as well as his brother. While behind bars, he has completed his college education by receiving a bachelor's degree. He helps other prisoners further their education and has been a model inmate. He works in the office of the minimum security prison.

In exchange for the promise of immunity from the death penalty, Heirens claims he was forced into confessing at age seventeen. Although the U.S. Court of Appeals and the Illinois Supreme Court agree that there were flagrant violations of Heirens rights, both continue to uphold the conviction *based on the confession*. After 56 years of incarceration Heirens is the longest serving inmate in Illinois history. He continues to maintain his innocence.

Student Profilers

Brettne Sanders PA, Anna Boswell, and Wanda Cox

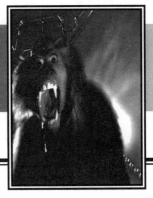

Aftermath

I. Word Scholar

Define the following words from *The Word Scholar Glossary.*

1. Nihilist _____

2. Sexual psychopathy _____

3. Antisocial parenting _____

4. "cool-coded" _____

5. Forensic neuropsychologist _____

6. Evolutionary neuroanatomy _____

7. "Serial" _____

8. "MO" _____

9. "Signature" _____

10. Serial killer _____

II. The Forensic Lab

Compose a one page report on the following: Discuss the similarities between "mild" and "moderate" psychopathy (see page 11) with the "Bad Boy" image in pop culture and Darwin's *survival of the fittest* notion of adaptability. If psychopaths really don't care about others except for novelty or sexual stimulation might psychopaths be more emotionally fit to survive?

CHAPTER 2

The "Narrow Down" Principle: Assessment & Profiling

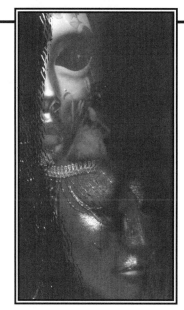

❝ . . ."*Experience has taught him to wait from four days to a week to harvest a hide. Sudden weight loss makes the hide looser and easier to remove. A stuporous resignation comes over some of them . . . it is necessary to provide a few rations to prevent despair and destructive tantrums . . .Tomorrow afternoon, he can do it . . .The next day at the latest. Soon.* **❞**

—*Silence of the Lambs*
Thomas Harris

"No two crimes or criminals are exactly alike. The profiler looks for patterns in the crimes and tries to come up with the characteristics of the likely offender. It's fact-based and uses analytical and logical thinking processes. We learn all we can from *what* happened, use our experience to fathom the probable reasons *why* it happened, and from these factors draw a *portrait of the perpetrator* of the crime; in a nutshell: What plus why equals who."

—Robert Ressler *(Whoever Fights Monsters)*

◼ Profiling Masquerade

The connotation of the word "profiling" is *au courant* in the field of violent crime investigation. As we have seen, criminal profiling produces a handy document as a "mousetrap" for a *special breed of violent criminals*, the true human predators of society: serial killers. Given crime scene evidence, the profile produces characteristics of the most likely suspect who is known initially as the UNSUB.

A rich history of the term "profiling" masquerading as "assessment" can be found in all forms of *clinical psychotherapy* stretching back as far as researchers want to go. To the Ph.D. psychologist (and MD-trained clinical psychiatrist), both profiling and assessment are *investigative tools* that seek to "narrow down" and uncover information. Assessment seeks to identify *clinical pathologies* (e.g. depression or personality disorders) through diagnosis and treatment **protocol**. Profiling seeks to identify the most likely UNSUB through "diagnosis" of the crime scene and offers a sketch of his behavioral and psychological proclivities.

However, a compelling argument can be made that accurate *pre-crime assessment* of psychopathic tendencies in the general population might preclude the necessity of post-crime profiling. Perhaps as a society, we stand on the brink of initiating preventive criminology. It may be, more than any other factor, the potentiality of daily intrusion into our lives by serial killers and adolescent "Rambo" killers that necessitate a tectonic shift in thinking. Only time will tell.

As we will discover, both **assessment** of suspected mental disorders in psychiatric patients who "present" symptoms in clinical interviews, as well as profilers who *profile* serial crimes from forensic evidence left behind at the crime scene, function to "narrow down" possible contingencies. Assessment to the clinician "narrows down" possible *psychological dysfunction* and *etiology* (causation) in patients suffering from anxiety, depression, or other pure psychopathologies; in contrast, profiling "narrows down" a match of *forensics* to one UNSUB—a sexual psychopath suggested by the *nature of the crime.*

The fact that behavior (*normal, dysfunctional,* or *criminal*) underlies personality is the guiding psychological principle that drives both assessment (in the clinical picture) and profiling (in the criminal picture). Both clinicians and profilers contend "behavior always gives them (clients and criminals) away."

◼ Domains of Information

Technically, what does it mean for clinicians or investigators to "assess" or "profile"? To the clinician, assessment refers to analyzing *dysfunctional behavior* observed or speculated upon as *presenting symptoms* in the clinical interview measured against *known pathological characteristics* in the reference "bible" of psychopathology, the DSM. (Like criminal profilers, clinicians rely on *inductive* methods—observed symptoms from patients used as "yardsticks" for measuring current "presenting symptoms", not mere deductive speculation of "what might be."

Clinicians seek to connect "presenting symptoms" of clients to other *domains of information* such as the **multiaxial system** of assessment in use by clinical psychologists. The *axial system* guards against accidental exclusion of vital clinical information.

In the DSM, for example, *Axis I* documents the existence of *pure psychopathologies,* such as depression and anxiety as clinical disorders.

Axis II documents *personality disorders* or *mental retardation*.

Axis III reports *general medical conditions* such as tumors or blood disorders.

Axis IV summarizes psychosocial and environmental problems such as divorce or emotional trauma upon the presenting symptoms of the patient.

Axis V reports the global assessment of functioning (GAF) scale—the general psychological condition of the client observable at any given time.

Axial information is necessary for the most comprehensive and professional diagnoses and treatment of clients so that all "bases" are covered.

◼ Profiling

Similarly, profiling "assesses" criminal evidence present at the crime scene "presented" by the nature of the **crime** and **victimology**—characteristics of the chosen victim. This information is compared to *known offender characteristics*—perpetrators who committed similar crimes.

Both the profiler and the clinician seek to *connect* their analyses to other *domains of information*. The criminal profiler (with laboratory help from forensic pathologists) seeks to connect the nature of the crime, victimology, and crime scene forensics to a specific perpetrator(s). On the other hand, the clinician attempts to untangle the neurochemical and societal influences contributing to a client's behavioral psychopathology.

The absolute necessity of connecting clinical information and criminal profiling to other domains of information relies on philosophical determinism. **Determinism** connects *cause and effect* to other domains of information as *cornerstones of science*. Determinism explains why the courtroom in violent crime cases has become a *theatre of forensics*. When effect is connected to cause, fact trumps speculation every time.

◼ Presenting Symptoms

To the clinician, a client's "presenting symptoms" sets up an assessment of personality influences, **milieu** influences, and possible chemical imbalances. Assessment leads directly to identifying disorders, dysfunction, maladaptive behavior, and neurochemical underpinnings. In fact, the *DSM* compiles or "profiles" mental and emotional disorders from observing characteristics of disorders across a wide continuum of influences that are indexed mild, moderate, or severe. For example, a "profile" exists for bipolarity, schizophrenia, or dissociative disorder in the DSM taxonomies. If clients "present" symptoms matching the "profile" listed in the clusters for personality disorders, for example, a clinical diagnosis is made.

Presenting symptoms "narrows down" diagnoses to an experienced clinician. In addition to a diagnosis, treatment protocols—such as talk therapy, prescriptive medications, and possible hospital commitment—are generated from DSM taxonomy. Similarly, a psychiatric social worker compiles a very useful tool, the psychosocial history assessment, which "profiles" family dynamics.

The psychosocial history documents a client's diagnosis by connecting it to other domains of information, such as:

1. Family history of dysfunction/addiction,
2. Communication patterns,
3. Lack of nurturing,
4. Personality disintegration, and
5. Societal and psychosocial influences.

Many of these *psychological influences* are of concern to criminal profilers as they meticulously piece together profiles of predators from crime scene evidence (similar to "presenting symptoms" of psychiatric patients).

■ Assessing Serial Killer Characteristics

From careful evaluation of paper-and-pencil inventories, face-to-face interviews, and crime scene evidence, profilers have uncovered the following general characteristics of serial killers.

Serial killers tend to be:

1. White males, 25–34 years of age,
2. Have an average IQ
3. Often possess charisma, or possess a charming personality (aka psychopathic)
4. Experienced abuse as children and/or were illegitimate
5. Select *specific types* of victims PEA.-Attracts people to a certain profile.
6. Select *vulnerable victims* they can control and dominate
7. Prefer to kill "hands on" such as strangulation and/or stabbing
8. Display *sexually sadistic fantasies*
9. Are impressed with police work and may impersonate officers as a ruse
10. Operate in all parts of North America with the higher incidence in southern states
11. Often have mental illness in family histories
12. Often have parents who have criminal backgrounds
13. Have a familial history of alcohol and/or drug abuse
14. Almost every one was subjected to *serious emotional abuse* during childhood
15. Are *sexually dysfunctional as adults*—no satisfying, mutually satisfying, give-and-take experience in mature sexual relationships

With few exceptions, serial killers are not psychotic, meaning at the time of the commission of the crime, they were not insane; as previously noted, they know exactly what they are doing. One notable exception is serial killer Richard Trenton Chase, the "Vampire of Sacramento".

PREDATOR PROFILE (2-1)

Richard Trenton Chase
"The Vampire of Sacramento"

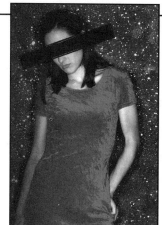

Span of Time Crimes Committed:

From December 29th, 1977 to late January, 1978, a total of 4 days.

Childhood:

Richard Trenton Chase was born on May 23, 1950. According to family reports, he was a mischievous child who grew up in a household of anger, mental illness, and alcoholism. Richard's mother was an alcoholic and a drug addict who displayed features of schizophrenia; his father was a compulsive disciplinarian who used physical abuse as a way to solve problems. As a child, Chase seemed to live in a fantasy world. Later, he became a fire-starter who showed no remorse.

As he grew older his crimes escalated to more serious offenses. He was a loner, showing signs of antisocial behavior. He was never perceived as a "ladies' man." He was ridiculed for being sexually impotent. Often he found dead animals, brought them home, and likely cannibalized them. Once, he injected rabbit blood into his veins, making him very ill. Eventually, psychiatrists diagnosed Chase with paranoid schizophrenia with features of somatic (bodily) delusions.

Physical Description of the Offender:

Chase was a white male 27 years of age, 5 ft. 11 inches tall, weighing approximately 145 lbs, appearing undernourished. He appeared as a homeless person with an unshaved beard, long brown hair, and sunken eyes.

Prior Offences to Serial Killings:

Most of his "priors" (prior offenses) were petty thefts, public intoxication, drinking while driving, possession of narcotics and resisting arrest. He was nothing more than a petty criminal. When he was arrested for carrying a gun without a license and torturing animals, soon thereafter the killing began.

Modus Operandi (MO):

Chase qualified as a *disorganized* killer. He walked from door to door checking to see which doors were unlocked. There was no planning involved. He believed if the door was locked you were "unwelcome." After finding an unlocked door, Chase entered with the intent to kill. When he found victims he would usually shoot them in the head and proceed to the next level of his sexualized crimes.

Known Signature:

Postmortem, Chase raped and mutilated the body of the women he killed. This mutilation extended far beyond overkill. Chase consumed human organs and drank victims' blood. On some occasions he extracted the organs and entrails to be consumed later. Often, Chase brought buckets with him to the crime scene. He filled them up with victims' blood.

Current Status:

Richard Chase was found dead in his cell on December 27, 1980 with enough medication in his body to kill three men. He committed suicide with a drug overdose.

Comments:

One of the few serial killers to suffer from mental illness, Chase believed he had a disease that turned his blood into powder, therefore giving rise to his *blood fetish*. He referred to his problem as "The Soap Dish Disease." In a fit of mania, Chase once ran through a hospital complaining that someone had stolen his organs. Chase remained unremorseful for his serial crimes.

Student Contributors:

Jeremy Crabb, Amanda Roderick, Brandon Strickland, Kimberly Bunt, and Heather Mitchell, PA

FBI: Fact or Fiction?

1. Within the FBI, *hostage negotiation* provided a steppingstone into criminal profiling since both procedures are interested in the criminal mind. **Fact or Fiction?**

2. The "softer" approach of hostage negotiation gained favor in the FBI in the 1980s over SWAT Team intervention, which evolved in the 1960s–1970s from Green Berets coming out of Vietnam. SWAT Teams receive special weapons and tactics (SWAT) training. **Fact or Fiction?**

3. The use of behavioral psychology goes beyond hostage negotiation and profiling by compiling databases of the *National Center for the Analysis of Violent Crime* and the *Violent Criminal Apprehension Program (VICAP),* the heart of the FBI's *inductive* method of hunting serial offenders. **Fact or Fiction?**

4. During the formative stages of developing protocols of criminal profiling, the FBI was *very interested* in what motivated murderers, rapists, and child molesters even though the offenses were not against federal laws. **Fact or Fiction?**

5. Murder is not a federal offense. **Fact or Fiction?**

6. Taking FBI courses on the road, known as "road shows," presented to local law enforcement agencies across the country allowed profilers to interview incarcerated serial offenders in remote locations. **Fact or Fiction?**

7. The "Stockholm syndrome" means a victim of crime *identifies with a captor* and places trust in him. **Fact or Fiction?**

8. *The Criminal Personality Research Project* (Ressler, 1970s) contributed nothing to criminal profiling. **Fact or Fiction?**

9. Interviewing violent criminals may cause some interviewers to develop *psychophysiological problems* (bleeding ulcers, hypertension, anxiety). **Fact or Fiction?**

10. Berkowitz *truly believed* his neighbor's dog was possessed by a 3,000-year old demon barking at him the orders to kill. **Fact or Fiction?**

11. Some murderers do in fact return to the scene of their crimes. **Fact or Fiction?**

12. Media coverage of serial killers can stimulate the offender to commit more crimes. **Fact or Fiction?**

13. The term "serial killer" was once referred to as "stranger killer." **Fact or Fiction?**

14. Serial killers are like Jeckle & Hyde—one minute they display normal behavior like Dr. Jeckle, and the next they're insane monsters like Mr. Hyde. **Fact or Fiction?**

15. According to Ressler, serial killers are obsessed with deviant fantasy and commit crimes that are essentially "non-fulfilling." **Fact or Fiction?**

SOURCE: *Whoever Fights Monsters* (Ressler, 1992).

■ Futuristic Application

A notable difference between clinicians and profilers is pre-crime versus post-crime analysis. In clinical assessment, the patient "presents" symptoms in real time, during therapy. In criminal profiling, the crime scene "speaks" to investigators and profilers who seek to reconstruct the events of the crime.

Suppose authorities could generate both a pre-crime *assessment* and a post-crime *profile* on serial killers such as a Ted Bundy typology, for example? It is not far-fetched to suggest that forensic psychologists (psychologists who testify on the validity and meaning of crime scene evidence in court) might be dumbstruck with psychological similarities between the two documents. In other words, effective *assessment* should indicate tendencies toward antisocial behavior. This could be validated by scores on a psychological **inventory test** such as the *Minnesota Multiphasic Personality Inventory (MMPI),* as well as a **projective test**, seeking the deeper dynamics of personality such as the *Thematic Apperception Test (TAT)* or *Rorschach Inkblots.* Pre-crime criminal assessment should accurately predict propensities for future criminal behavior, at least so goes the theory.

Speculatively, will there ever be a time when forensic psychologists, acting as "behavioral police" intervene (in pre-crime) with an assessment analysis to arrest future expression of crime? This notion was presented recently in Stephen Spielberg's *Minority Report* as the Department of Pre-Crime. If authorities are 99% sure an individual has the *requisite psychopathic personality* and neurological damage to commit murder, rape, or serial crime, why would authorities hesitate to intercede before the act of murder or rape is accomplished?

This is precisely what happens in profiling once a particular crime is connected to a targeted offender. Authorities seek to arrest the suspect with a search and/or arrest warrant. *Why not intervene before the death of innocent victims?*

As a preventive measure, might all citizens of the United States eventually be required to be assessed for *criminal tendencies* using a profiler's "pre-crime assessment"? To the **futurist**, might this document be required prior to the issuance of a driver's license or required on a person's twenty-first birthday? Might this assessment prevent crime and the need of a criminal profile? Due to the reorganization of the FBI's focus on terrorism with less time devoted to serial crimes, might the timing be right to consider "pre-crime" assessment? Would a Department of Pre-Crime within the Department of Justice impinge upon our constitutional rights? If citizens were required to answer an inventory of criminal tendencies, might it resemble the questionnaire developed by our criminal profiling students?

■ From the Desk of Student Criminal Profilers—Targeting Psychopathy

Pre-Crime Assessment Questionnaire

1. Have you ever "acted out" by hitting or harming another person? No. Yes. If yes, under what circumstances? Explain. Recently, have you had thoughts of harming another? If yes, explain.
2. Are you currently taking prescribed medication? For what medical/ psychological condition? Discuss any and all mental illness in your immediate family.
3. Do you agree or disagree: I do not feel compelled to always live by the rules of society. Explain.
4. Have you ever had an incident of road rage where you were the attacker? Explain.
5. Have you ever been diagnosed with a mental or emotional disorder? Have you ever been an inmate of a psychiatric hospital? No. Yes. Explain.
6. On a scale of 1–10 (with 10 being the highest), to what degree to you value your life and the lives of others? Explain.
7. On a scale of 1–10 (10 being the highest), how active is your fantasy life? Give two examples of your sexual fantasies. Do you believe any of your fantasies are deviant?
8. Do you harbor animosities against individuals with different ethnicities/race/ or gender other than yours? Explain.
9. Have you ever been arrested? No. Yes. Explain.
10. Are you quick to anger? No. Yes. Explain.
11. Are you currently registered as a sexual offender? No. Yes. For what offense?
12. Were you abused (sexually, verbally, or physically) as a child? No. Yes. Explain.
13. Has a court ever required mandatory attendance for you at an anger management class? No. Yes. Explain.
14. What is your opinion of men who hit women? What is your opinion of serial rapists and serial killers?

■ What's Eating Jack?

Returning to our analysis of the words "profiling" versus "assessment," when the word "criminal" or the words "violent crime" are added to the word "profiling" we get the connotation the FBI had in mind when developing the criminal profile. The difference is considerable and moves criminal profiling closer to the auspices of criminal justice and criminology. Popular culture provides a helpful analogy in the perception of a fictional character Jack Torrance from the novel *The Shining* by Stephen King.

> "Jack Torrance picks up the ax and buries it in the chest of Dick Hollorann."

Frustrated novelist Jack Torrance takes his psychological pathologies a step further by killing an Overlook Hotel employee and then stalking with an ax his own wife, Wendy, and son, Danny. Had Jack escaped the snowbound lodge, he would be a fitting subject for criminal profiling. Had he not committed criminal offenses—one homicide and two attempted murders—his behavior would have remained non-criminal, although admittedly pathologically unstable and need of assessment, diagnosis, and treatment.

It's a scary thought that many individuals in society are "Jack Torrances"—slowly "simmering" in sexual psychopathy, yet remaining undiagnosed. They are functional "dysfunctionals," much like we observe in functional alcoholics, individuals who remain productive, psychosocially, with addiction to alcohol.

◼ *Corpus Delicti—Mens Rea, Actus Reus, and the Corpse*

Criminal perpetrators "act out" by going beyond the cognitive component of crime—the legalistic concept of *criminal mental intent* known as **mens rea**—literally "guilty mind." In doing so, criminals cross the invisible line between "thinking about it" and "acting out" with a criminal act—the physical part of the crime known as **actus reus**—literally "guilty action."

Both *mens rea* (mental) and *actus reus* (physical) comprise what criminal attorneys recognize as elements of *corpus delicti*—the *body of evidence* prosecuting attorneys need to win their case. (Interestingly, *corpus delicti* is often misrepresented in **pop culture** especially in movies as "the body of the dead victim," which is not true.) *Corpus delicti* refers to *rules of evidence* regarding the mental state of intent as it merges with the physical act, producing the dead victim. Both *mens rea* and *actus reus* will be further investigated as elements of *modus vivendi*—the sexualized elements of serial crimes—in Chapter Five.

◼ Severity of Rapacious Behavior

In the case of the serial criminal, no treatment exists to reverse his rapacious behavior. This is not because the person is just "bad" or "evil." The reason in most cases is due to *horrific abuses from antisocial parenting* that produces *irreversible neurological brain damage*. What else would explain their blatant disregard for human life? Due to damaged brains, they perceive the world far differently than a person with a normal brain. Every serial killer must be incarcerated for life with no possibility of parole or face capital punishment. Once serial killers "get a taste" of rapacious crime, they are driven to commit more offenses. Serial killers never commit suicide unless cornered by authorities with no hope of escape. Obviously *self-aware* of their heinous acts, they choose to end their own cowardly lives exemplified by Andrew Cunanan following the murder of fashion designer Gianni Versace.

◼ Narcissism

Many serial killers possess features of *narcissistic personality disorder*. Suicide is entirely out of the question when perpetrators display **narcissistic** traits as observed in the opinion of Charles Manson's former prosecuting attorney Vincent Bugilosi in his book *Outrage*. In the book, Bugilosi recounts the O. J. Simpson trial. Convinced of Simpson's guilt and **narcissistic personality disorder,** he correctly observed (as did other forensic psychologists) that Simpson would not harm himself and would have never shot himself in the now famous LA freeway "chase." Almost to the man, serial killers (of the organized typology) are narcissistic, arrogant, and believe that they are intellectually superior to pursuers.

Psychiatric patients with psychological dysfunction are assessed in an effort to recapture mental and emotional health focusing on *liberation and regaining self-esteem and respect*. Criminals must be incarcerated or "warehoused" in prisons, while psychologically dysfunctional individuals seek liberation from their self-imposed emotional "prisons."

◼ Profiling: Connection Between Autopsies and Psychology

As we have seen, the Atlanta child murders provided the launch pad for media and law enforcement scrutiny of the criminal profile, but, lost in the archives of time, contemporary historians cannot agree on the date of the first criminal profile. However, the tortured minds of killers have been brilliantly displayed in many works of literature since recorded history. Cain and Able from the Old Testament, or perhaps, as a group, the tragedies of Shakespeare best exemplify how a tortured mind like Othello, for example, is driven to murder his wife. Or, the science fiction novels of Sir Arthur Canon Doyle recount the many puzzle pieces detective Sherlock Holmes and Dr. Watson pieced together in their efforts to identify criminals. Using his magnifying glass and collection of chemicals, Holmes even had a functional forensic lab in his Baker Street residence.

Outside of science fiction, could autopsies have provided the initial setting for criminal profiling? Some investigators suggest this possibility by pointing to the postmortem exam performed by Dr. Thomas Bond, M.D., a police surgeon, on Mary Kelly, the last victim of Jack the Ripper. Suggested by wound patterns, Dr. Bond surmised other victims fit the pattern of the killer's *modus operandi* (MO). Today, MO—the killer's "operational methods,"—and "signature,"—what *fulfills his sexual and psychological needs* and links murders to the same perpetrator—was personified in the Ripper crimes.

However, not all profiles are the results of physical evidence gathered at crime scenes or postmortem exams. World War II provided an example of profiling a war criminal and mass murder. A psychiatrist, Dr. Walter Langer, was asked by the CIA to provide a profile of Adolph Hitler.

Since it was unrealistic to assume Hitler would die of natural causes or be caught alive, the essence of the profile focused on "what made him tick." (In the unlikely event Hitler was captured alive, the profile suggested ways to interrogate him, a common practice today.) Langer's profile suggested Hitler saw himself as "savior of his country" and if his capture seemed certain, he would commit suicide, which actually occurred. Today, it is common practice in law enforcement to profile leaders of *military campaigns* and those who claim responsibility for *terrorist attacks*.

Profilers Seek Answers Beyond Persona

The following is a list of pertinent questions a profiler seeks to answer:

1. What are his behavioral and psychological characteristics?
2. Based on the nature of the crime (related to MO and signature), what makes him tick?
3. What might be some of his most recognizable physical characteristics? Based upon what the crime scene suggests did he have to carry the victim from place to place? Is he physically strong or weak?
4. By the nature of the crime, what are his fantasies? Sadistic? Sexually perverse?
5. What did he leave behind relative to psychosocial influences that seem at work on his tortured psyche?
6. Where does he live?
7. Where kind of work might he perform? Regarding the time of the murder, is he a shift worker? Did he leave any evidence from his shoes or clothing that suggests his line of work?

Fact or Fiction?

Whoever Fights Monsters
A True Crime Book

By Robert Ressler

1. According to Ressler, serial killers *have control over their emotions,* allowing them to avoid detection (versus being out of control) so that *truth serum* and *lie detectors* are useless because they can "beat" them. **Fact or Fiction?**

2. Profilers look for patterns in crimes and try to deduce characteristics of the offender from fact-based data in the FBI supercomputers so that "*what* plus *why* equals *who*." **Fact or Fiction?**

3. What profilers call a "rape kit" refers to what forensic specialists bring to the crime scene to gather evidence against the perpetrator. **Fact or Fiction?**

4. A mentally ill killer never ranges far from home in seeking victims. **Fact or Fiction?**

5. A *forensic odontologist* can match bite marks on a victim to a perpetrator. **Fact or Fiction?**

6. According to Ressler, *unlimited sexual experimentation* is not a category of behavior observed in serial killers. **Fact or Fiction?**

7. A lie detector does not detect lies; rather it *detects fear* through physiological changes in the body (such as heart rate, blood pressure, and breathing). **Fact or Fiction?**

8. "Truth serum" is actually *sodium pentothal* and does not make anyone tell the truth or cause anyone to lose control. It is a short-acting barbiturate (sedative) that produces general anesthesia, relaxation, and a susceptibility to suggestion. It is a misnomer to suggest it makes a person "tell the truth." **Fact or Fiction?**

9. Manson family members were blood related except for Charles "Tex" Watson. **Fact or Fiction?**

10. Bundy's final attempt to "con" and manipulate authorities occurred when he invited Dr. James Dobson to interview him prior to being executed the next morning. **Fact or Fiction?**

SOURCE: *Whoever Fights Monsters* (Ressler, 1992).

ANSWERS: 1. Fact 2. Fact 3. Fiction 4. Fact 5. Fact 6. Fiction 7. Fact 8. Fact 9. Fiction 10. Fact

PREDATOR PROFILE (2-2)

Ed Gein
"The Plainfield Ghoul"

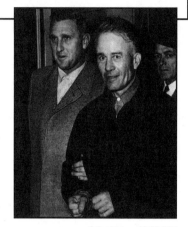
©Bettmann/CORBIS

Introduction

This profile is based on true-life serial killer Ed Gein. Born on a farm and raised by a domineering mother, in the space of a few years his entire family died, leaving him alone as caretaker of the family farm. In the next few years, the dark side of Ed Gein came out—he became a grave robber, a necrophiliac, and a cannibal. In the most perverted twist of any serial killer, he became a demonic "artist" by crafting body parts into "artwork." Ed Gein is the most bizarre serial killer of the twentieth century, perhaps even more perverted than the serial killer and cannibal Jeffrey Dahmer. Gein's crimes inspired the movies *Psycho, The Texas Chainsaw Massacre* and *Silence of the Lambs*.

Alternative Media Monikers:

"The Butcher of Plainfield"
"The Mad Butcher"

DOB/DOD:

Born 1906, died July, 1984.

Residence (at time of murders):

160-acre farm seven miles outside Plainfield, Wisconsin.

Types of Crimes:

Serial killer, grave robber, necrophiliac, cannibalism, sadism, and death fetish.

Weapons Used:

.22 rifle & .32 revolver

Victim Vicinity:

Plainfield, Wisconsin

Murder Time Span:

1954 to 1957

Victim Typology:

Older Women; motherly types

In the Beginning

Ed Gein and his brother Henry were raised by a domineering mother who was a religious fanatic obsessed with her boys avoiding women, the main constituent of sin, in her view. She discouraged her boys from even looking at women. She kept them busy with farm work from dusk until dawn. Ed's alcoholic father died in 1940 and a few years later his brother Henry died, allegedly trapped while fighting a forest fire.

Shortly thereafter, his mother suffered her first stroke. In 1945 she had her second stroke from which she never recovered. Ed was left alone.

At this point, he sealed off the upstairs, the parlor, and his mother's bedroom and set up his own quarters in the remaining bedroom, kitchen and shed of the farmhouse. He stopped working the farm because a government soil-conservation program offered him a tidy subsidy, which he augmented by his work as a handyman.

The Graveyard

In his spare time Ed read books on human anatomy and Nazi concentration camp experiments. He became obsessed with the photos, especially the sections dealing with female anatomy. Alone in the farmhouse, he obsessed about sex, the subject so detested and repressed in young Ed by his mother. One day he saw a newspaper report of a woman who had been buried that day. He enlisted the help of friend, a loner named Gus, to help him rob his first grave, ostensibly for "medical experiments."

The first corpse came from a grave very close to the final resting place of Gein's mother. Over the next several years, Gein checked the newspaper for newly buried bodies, always visiting the graveyard at the time of a full moon. At times, he stole the entire corpse of dead females, or at other times, just the parts he wanted.

Corpse "experiments" included constructing objects from the bones and skin of corpses, such as furniture and purses. He stored organs in his refrigerator to consume later. He also committed acts of necrophilia—sex with the dead bodies. He even dug up his own mother's corpse.

Gein never revealed to anyone his growing desire to become a woman himself. This transgender obsession ended with his construction of a full female "bodysuit" complete with death mask and breasts constructed entirely of human skin. When Gus, his co-conspirator and grave robber, was taken away to the lunatic asylum, Ed found himself alone again. Leaving grave robbing behind, Ed turned to serial murder for live bodies.

The Murders

Gein's first victim was Mary Hogan, a 51-year-old divorcee who operated Hogan's Tavern at Pine Grove, six miles from his home. She was alone when he came to her on the cold afternoon of 8 December 1954. He shot her in the head with his 32-caliber revolver, placed her body in his pickup truck, and took her back to his farmhouse shed.

A would-be customer found the tavern deserted and a large bloodstain on the floor. He noticed a spent .32 cartridge near the bloodstain that led out the back door and into the parking lot. From all appearances, it looked as if Mary Hogan had been shot and taken away. Police were unable to find any clues to the disappearance. A few weeks later when a sawmill owner spoke of the disappearance to Gein he replied: "She isn't missing. She's at the farm right now." And that was that.

There may have been other victims in the years that followed, but nothing definite is known about Gein's murderous activities until November 1957, when Gein shot and killed Bernice Worden in her hardware store on Plainfield's Main Street. He used a .22 rifle from a display rack in the store, inserting his own bullet, which he carried with him. Gein removed her body and locked the store, taking the body home in the pickup owned by the hardware store.

Ms. Worden's son, Frank, often assisted her in the store, but on this particular Saturday morning he'd gone deer hunting. When he returned in the late afternoon he discovered the store closed with the lights on and his mother missing. There was blood on the floor.

A local garage attendant told him that he had seen the store truck driving away at about 9.30 A.M. that morning. Since Frank Worden served as deputy sheriff in the area he immediately alerted the sheriff. He checked the record of sales transactions made that morning and discovered one for a half-gallon of antifreeze. Worden remembered that Ed Gein had stopped by the previous evening at closing time and said he'd be back the next morning for antifreeze. Ed had also asked Worden if he intended to go hunting the next day. Since the cash register was missing, it appeared that Gein had planned a robbery after finding a suitable time when the coast would be clear. Worden told of his suspicions to the sheriff. The sheriff and captain of the local PD set off for the farm, seven miles outside Plainfield.

Arriving at Gein's house they found it uninhabited and dark. Acting on a hunch, they drove to a store in West Plainfield where Gein usually purchased groceries. They caught him just as he was leaving. They detained him for questioning. Gein told the lawmen he believed someone had tried to frame him for Bernice Worden's death. Immediately, he was taken into custody since no one knew of Ms. Worden's death.

The officers returned to his farmhouse. The doors to the farmhouse were locked, but the door to the side shed at the rear of the house was open. Since the farmhouse had no electricity, the sheriff had to use a torch to see. What they found was horrific! The wall of the shed revealed a naked corpse of a woman hanging upside down from a crossbeam, the legs spread wide apart, and a long slit running from the genitals almost to the throat. But the throat, like the head, was missing. The genitals and the anus had been cut out. Bernice Worden had been disemboweled as though preparing a deer for processing.

Human Trophies

Looking further, the shed and the farmhouse appeared as though it had not been cleaned in many years as piles of rubbish were everywhere. The few rooms that weren't barricaded were littered with piles of junk. Amid the junk, officers found the following human remains:

1. two shin bones,
2. four human noses,
3. an empty quart can converted into a tom-tom by human skin stretched over both top and bottom,
4. a bowl made from the inverted half of a human skull,
5. nine death masks (from the well-preserved skin from the faces of women),
6. ten female heads with the tops sawn off above the eyebrows,
7. bracelets of human skin,
8. a purse made with a handle of human skin,
9. a sheath for a knife made in human skin,
10. a pair of leggings made from human skin,
11. four chairs with the seats being replaced by strips of human skin,
12. a shoe box containing nine salted vulvas of which his mother's was painted silver,
13. a hanging human head,
14. a lampshade covered with human skin,
15. a shirt made of human skin,
16. a number of shrunken heads (Ed always joked that he had a collection of shrunken heads),
17. two skulls for Gein's bedposts,
18. a pair of human lips hanging from string,

19. Ed's full woman body suit constructed with human skin and complete with mask and breasts,
20. Bernice Worden's heart in a pan on the stove, and
21. human organs stacked in the refrigerator

The bodies of 15 different women had been mutilated to provide Gein's "artistic" trophies. Rumor had it that Gein often brought gifts of fresh venison to his neighbors although it was well known that Gein had never shot a deer in his life.

Upon capture, Gein received a series of examinations at the Central State Hospital for the Criminally Insane. He was proven insane. Examiners believed he both loved and hated his mother; this emotional ambivalence proved to be the trigger that drove him to kill older women and eventually into insanity. Many believed Mary Hogan had more than a passing resemblance to his mother.

The case created a sensation because of the true nature of the crime. Thousands of people drove to Plainfield to get a look at the "murder farm." Eventually, the Plainfield citizens burned down the Gein farmhouse as they regarded it as a "place of evil." On Christmas day 1957, Gein was judged insane and he was committed to Waupun State Hospital for the rest of is life. Gein died of cancer in 1984, at the age of 78. He was buried in Plainfield next to the graves of his family.

Possible victims of Gein are an eight-year-old girl who went missing in 1947 and a fifteen-year-old girl who had disappeared on her way home from babysitting in 1953. The babysitter's bloodstained clothes were found but no body. In Ed's house there were plenty of body parts, which did not come from his grave robbing or two known murders.

The Movies

Ed Gein's bizarre victimization of women inspired the literature and film industry. Because of the true nature of his crimes it gave Hollywood surreal material. One early film was Alfred Hitchcock's *Psycho* based on the Robert Bloch novel. The connection being Norman Bates' overpowering mother and the horror of the film, made Psycho an instant classic. *The Texas Chainsaw Massacre* is another film based on Gein. The story is about a group of traveling teens that stumble on a "horror house" of weird homicidal cannibals—the lead weirdo is Leatherface—who robbs graves and constructs furniture made of bones and skulls. Leatherface gets "jazzed" by chasing teens around with his chainsaw and wearing the human death masks of his victims.

The final film is the Academy Award winning movie *Silence of the Lambs*. It's about an FBI agent who's tracking down a serial killer, and to find him she must get the help of an intelligent cannibal, Dr. Hannibal Lector. The serial killer she's trying to track down is called 'Buffalo Bill' because he secretly wants to be a woman. He kills women to make a "girl suit" out of their skin.

Conclusion

Technically, Ed Gein was not a serial killer since he only killed two women. Yet, he remains a suspect in the disappearance of others, but the "museum of horrors" found at his farmhouse definitely made him infamous as the most bizarre killer in history.

Contributed By:

Cherie Ellis, criminal profiling student

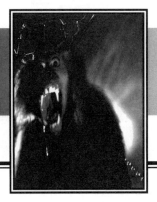

Aftermath

I. Word Scholar

Define the following words from *The Word Scholar Glossary*.

1. Assessment _____

2. Profiling _____

3. Determinism _____

4. *Corpus Delicti* _____

5. *Mens Rea* _____

6. *Actus Reus* _____

7. Pop culture _____

8. Milieu _____

9. Multiaxial System _____

10. Narcissistic Personality Disorder _____

II. The Forensic Lab

Compose a one page report on the following: What is your idea for determining severe forms of psychopathy before a person is granted a driver's license? Will brain scans be required by schools in the near future (just as vaccine records are now required)?

CHAPTER 3

Paradigms of Criminality

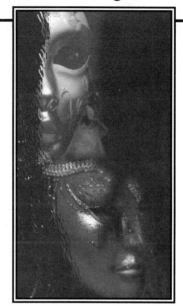

> ❝*The problem of killing this one had perplexed Mr. Gumb for days. Hanging her was out because he didn't want pectoral mottling, and besides, he couldn't risk the knot tearing her behind the ear . . . One cardinal principle: no matter how weak from hunger or faint with fright, they always fought you when they saw the apparatus . . .*❞

—*Silence of the Lambs*
Thomas Harris

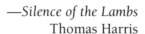

"Crime is the result of some *personality attribute* uniquely possessed, or possessed to a certain degree, by the potential criminal."

—Neitzel (1979)

◾ Systemic Knowledge of Crime

A paradigm is a philosophical, scientific, or criminological framework of systemic information complete with *intellectual rationale* to support *perspective* and *methodology. Paradigms organize information.* Nosology and taxonomy are two paradigmatic strategies for organization and analysis of information. For example, **nosology** refers to passages or chapters in a book written to define, describe, compare, and contrast terms on any given subject for purposes of illumination distilled into lists or categories. The end result of this intellectual (and often empirical) process results in **taxonomy**—a handy table or typology of influences, components, elements in chart form. (In chemistry, the *Periodic Table of Elements* is a well-known taxonomic chart. In pedagogy, *Bloom's Taxonomy* reveals the best ways to teach for student comprehension). Similar to most textbooks and reference books, the *DSM*, the principle diagnostic tool of clinical psychology and psychiatry, utilizes both nosology and taxonomy, as does this text.

Hence, a *criminological paradigm* is an attempt to provide systematized rationale for criminal behavior after theorizing, statistical analysis, and/or evidence gathering. For serial crime, the task is a daunting one considering the *sexualized pathology* observed in the sexual psychopathy. Serial killers comprise a special category of *sexual deviates* whose motive is born of lust-fantasy, sexual experimentation, and murder. The causes are varied, complex, and multi-layered. Save the unlikely possibility of discovering a "sexual psychopathy gene," *no single root cause exists.*

In targeting criminal behavior, including the violent, sexualized psychopath, researchers create paradigms—scientific "frameworks" for the creation of hypotheses and methodologies needed to systematically catalog knowledge. Always behind paradigmatic psychopathy is "what makes the sexual psychopath tick." To this end, it is necessary to restate our **operational definition** of *sexual psychopathy*. In our view, sexual psychopathy refers to sexually perverted personality and behavioral characteristics (Freud would call them "character flaws") evidenced by an antisocial personality disorder (DSM taxonomy) that compels a person to sequentially rape or murder others. In our view, the DSM is too non-descript and non-specific in categorizing serial killers as individuals with antisocial personality disorder. Yes, they are antisocial, but they are much, much more.

Sexual psychopaths characterize the sexual crimes perpetrated by serial killers.

Organized serial killers display a **glib**, superficial charm and engaging personality, yet underneath the well-crafted persona, they are unremorseful, insincere, deceitful, emotionally shallow, arrogant, and pathological liars. They display an uncaring attitude toward the welfare of others.

The salient familial features contributing to sexual psychopathy are horrific parental abuse (physical and/or sexual), and later, an addiction to hardcore pornography or similar erotic material further exacerbating deviant cognitive mapping. Due to the violence exhibited at crime scenes, the majority, if not all sexual psychopaths, display *irreversible neurological brain damage* exemplified by "cool-coded" brain scans.

The lethal mix of all three components—physical/sexual abuse, poly-addiction, and neuropathy—place the psychopath in a *special class of sexually deviant, violent criminals* whose behavior is considered incorrigible.

In molding psychopathic personality, incompetent and hateful **antisocial parenting** takes place in any number of parental abuses—verbal, physical, or sexual, neglect, lack of feelings promoting emotional bonding, lack of tender emotions or love, and/or feeling emotionally disconnected from the family. As a consequence, young "becoming" psychopaths feel bitterness, frustration, and ultimately rage for being "different." This deviant feeling partially explains why young psychopaths display the "red flags" of lack of control and aggression by becoming oppositional defiant by age 10 or sooner.

Both criminal and non-criminal psychopaths are consumed by *egocentricity*. Non-criminal psychopaths talk about themselves continually and tell others they have a lot of "confidence" or "arrogance" but that's "just the way I'm am." This is often calculated to impress female "targets" that seemed to be impressed by such things. Also, non-criminal psychopaths are quick to "laugh off" early criticism from a "targeted" victim—

a female he can emotionally and sexually "vandalize". He wants to show her how emotionally resilient he is so that "nothing bothers him." He wants her to known he feels invincible, yet another ploy for a victim with low self-esteem.

◼ Beware of "Bad Boy" Persona—"Mild" and "Moderate" Psychopaths

In the end, the victims of psychopaths, whether raped, murdered, fired from a job, or emotionally "ripped off," are the big losers. The emotional damage is often long lasting to inexperienced and immature females who are attracted to the psychopath's energy, daring, and *faux* romanticism. Females with low self-esteem can become addicted to psychopaths like a drug; they are often driven to please them long after the psychopath has lost interest. And, he always loses interest. For females who lack perspective, the "mild" to "moderate" psychopath are usually not killers, but they might engage in date rape, or shatter another life when they decide to move on. And they always move on to the "greener pastures" of a new sexual challenge. Sexual variety is their "spice of life." They want to feel, to savor, every sexual conquest to the fullest. They expect females to use birth control since a condom reduces his pleasure. He "walks" or tells her "it's your problem," or "I'll take care of it," but never does when she tells him "I'm late" (for her period). According to researcher H. Niborg, "He may be a good lover, but a very poor choice for a life long mate. He soon tires of the female he's with . . . she doesn't excite him anymore . . . so he moves on."

Adolescent psychopaths are incapable of forming long-standing, enduring relationships with others so that people are reduced to objects. Physiologically, some of these violence-prone adolescents show evidence of *lower thresholds of arousal* in the (ANS) autonomic nervous system, reinforcing one hypothesis requiring *extreme measures* to feel stimulated. Today, cognitive neuroscience and neuropsychology have compelling evidence of the "fractured" brains of violent criminals. The neuroscience of serial violence has a commanding presence in courtrooms today. It has not always been that way as a brief history lesson on the strides made by neuropsychology and forensic psychology will disclose.

◼ Pre-scientific Explanations of Crime— The Spirit World

Regardless of severity, criminals are individuals who commit crimes against the settled order of society. They are not law-abiding citizens who try to make communities safe. Through deception, deceit, and manipulation, criminals seek alternative ways of obtaining what they want over law-abiding citizens. The question is always why?

Historically, a millennium before the terms serial killer, mass murderer, or spree killers were invented, theories existed to explain why some individuals go down darker paths. As we have seen, sexual psychopaths (serial killers) are a breed apart from all other criminals. After a brief look at law and order versus criminality, we will address, neurochemically, why human predators are unique.

Despite Greek **humanism** in the 6th–8th century BC, the prevailing view of criminality and crimes in ancient times, and including the thousand years of the Dark Ages, revolved around superstition, demonology, witchcraft, and exorcism. Interestingly, the same criteria were often used for determining insanity.

In the sixteenth century, Paracelsus insisted that mental disorders had *natural causes* leading some scholars to consider criminal behavior in a similar light. Could criminal behavior have natural causes?

The oldest form of spiritual belief, **animism**—the belief that inanimate, as well as animate, objects in nature possess a spirit—was not too far removed from the folklore of shape shifting werewolves and demons of the seventeenth century *zeitgeist*. In the spirit world, *malevolent spirits* (such as Satan, witches, devils, and demons) take over, or "possess" a person causing them to do unspeakable evil as observed in the *Salem Witch Trials* (1492) in Salem, Mass. Hence, malevolent spirits and demon-spawned monsters "possessed" hapless humans to commit murder and other heinous acts. The modern Catholic belief in **exorcism** is an example of being purged from demon "possession" of a malevolent being.

In this malevolent spirit view, criminality came from outside sources—demons and devils—causing a person "to be possessed." The Biblical Satan is a logical choice for most demon possessions. During this time, French dream interpreters recognized "dwarf devils"—referred to as *chaucemar*—or "pressing devils," who sat upon the chest of dreamers causing nightmares.

In the late nineteenth century and early twentieth century aided by the Enlightenment and rationalism, early criminologists put criminal behavior squarely in the hands of the individuals who committed the crimes, not demon-possessed werewolves, witches, or malevolent spirits. Earlier with philosophical **rationalism**, and later with **humanistic psychology** (1960s), if a person could reach for the stars and catch a few, he might also stoop to the deepest forms of depravity.

Soon the *zeitgeist* changed to rational explanations, so that spirits were "out" and personal choices were "in." *Choices* and a strong dose of *personal responsibility* entered the formula of human behavior and provided a springboard to understanding the criminal mind. Investigators ask: "what makes up criminal personality (or criminal mind)?"

Not until the twentieth century did scientific researchers want to know the causes of serial homicides observed in *apparently motiveless crimes of sexual lust, mutilation, and murder committed against strangers.* The murders of Jack the Ripper had pointed the way to serial homicide several years earlier (1888).

◼ Mental Deficiency

In the twentieth century, some medical researchers theorized *mental deficiency* as a cause of criminal behavior. For example, a genetic disorder known as *Kleinfelter's Syndrome* was theorized to produce an aggressive criminal—a male with testicular malfunction and a bad complexion (due to acne). The birth defect was due to an extra X chromosome, the chromosomal sex being configured as XXY instead of the normal XY. This configuration resulted in a lower IQ, infertility (no viable sperm) and some degree of mental retardation. Some males with XXY were indeed aggressive but not criminal. (Today, the syndrome occurs in about 1 in 500 males.) While some criminals inherited the genetic disorder (for example, Richard Speck, mass murderer of eight student nurses in Chicago, was diagnosed with *Kleinfelter's Syndrome*), no direct evidence linked XXY to criminality for certainty; hence, the theory soon fell out of favor.

Interestingly, today, **ADD (Attention Deficit Disorder)** is often observed in individuals diagnosed as *oppositional defiant*. By no means do all oppositional defiant adolescents become sexual psychopaths. No serious researcher is prepared to content that *ADD* or its twin diagnostic "brother" **ADHD (Attention Deficit Hyperactivity Disorder)** actually causes criminality, although it may be a salient factor among many other psychosocial factors. It should come as no surprise that more boys than girls are diagnosed with ADD, ADHD, and oppositional defiance. A *testosterone hypothesis* has been advanced for this gender difference.

◼ Criminal Personality Traits

So far, a list of *criminal personality traits* has eluded investigators probably because no such hard-and-fast taxonomy exists. Criminalists remind us that the criminal is first an *individual with his own set of influences, habits, parenting, and brain chemistry*. Casual observers may ask: "Are not all serial killers 'defiant, hostile, and destructive'?" The answer is "Yes", but how they got that way depends on a variety of factors and requires more information. Researchers are hesitant to reduce *rapacious behavior* to singular psychosocial influences, or to biology alone.

Apparently remorseless, the sexual psychopath (or *sociopath* as preferred in sociology), acts without conscience, ignores the consequences of violence, and becomes a pawn to his own twisted sexual fantasies. He feels *compelled* to "act out" to assuage (pacify) sexual desires that continue to fuel perverted behavior. Forensic psychologists insist the criminal mind of psychopathy is far too complex and disordered to concoct an irrefutable checklist for rapacity. The forensic psychiatrists and psychologists always attempt to dig deeper into the human **psyche** (the root word for psychology, originally meaning "soul"). However, once a sexual psychopath, always a sexual psychopath as the "brutal urge" to rape and kill others extends well into predators who are over fifty years of age, long after testosterone has peaked.

A Medical Paradigm

Some psychiatrists suggest psychopathy may be due to one or more of the following factors:

1. Major neurological glitches in the Central Nervous System (CNS), especially in the emotional centers (mid-brain) and cerebellum,
2. Organic brain damage,
3. Severe chemical imbalances resulting from physical trauma, chronic malnutrition, and/or substance abuse,
4. Depersonalization (almost complete absence of self) brought about by negative or non-existent parenting, and/or sexual abuse issues,
5. Violent temper with no regard for social consequences, and/or
6. Vivid, sexual obsessions that provide focus and motivation to behavior.

◾ Paradigm of the Homicidal Triad

According to experienced profilers, the so-called **homicidal triad** is commonly observed in sexual psychopathy. This behavioral triad indicates "red flags," the potential ability for violent crimes, *showing lack of restraint* and a tendency to "act out." A *cavalier distain for structure and responsibility* is inherent in the triad, which includes:

1. **Enuresis** (en-yur-e-sis) or "bed wetting" at an inappropriate age,
2. **Cruelty to small children** (animals or pets), and
3. **Pyromania** (fire starting)

Besides low self-esteem, anger, frustration, and blaming others for severe childhood abuses and/or neglect, many serial predators (sexual psychopaths) have frightening histories of *compulsivity and ritualism such as lying, cheating, and compulsive masturbation.* As they enter late adolescence, they begin to display criminal "careers" as pyromaniacs, cat burglars, stalkers, Peeping Toms, rapists, and fetishism, before eventually (in their early to mid-twenties) committing murder.

◾ Neurochemical Paradigm: Testosterone Hypothesis

Testosterone is a genuine **aphrodisiac** responsible for sexual fantasy and behavior in both male and female. It is also the hormone responsible for aggression. Not surprisingly, studies in physiological psychology, medicine, and criminology consistently show elevated levels of testosterone correlates with high crime rates.

Libido can be a good thing, but apparently, it can get out of hand. The **androgenic** hormone testosterone not only lies behind libido, it also lies behind aggression and violence.

Compelling research regarding the powerful affects/effects of testosterone indicate a male with high testosterone may be a terrific lover, but a very poor choice for a long-term mate and role model for children. His need for sexual conquest and variety is overwhelming. Given other factors (soon to be defined), he may also be a killer when an inhibitory neurotransmitter serotonin (5-HT) is in scarce supply in the brain.

With surging levels of testosterone, some adolescent and young adult males seek sexual favors from a variety of females. They show extreme difficulty being loyal to just one mate. Apparently for some "high octane" males, one female is simply not enough to satisfy his ubiquitous sexual proclivities. Over-the-top levels of testosterone may account for why some males are so aggressive—by getting into fights and committing other criminal acts—especially when exacerbated by drugs or alcohol.

It is well known that in some males, alcohol consumption causes a drastic drop in serotonin levels, which may account for escalation of violence, whether in a barroom brawl or alone with a female when he can exercise complete control.

Sadly, with volumes of research regarding the effects of alcohol consumption (or other drugs) by males with high testosterone levels, law enforcement cannot intercede until he threatens injury or kills someone.

Other than advocacy programs such as *MADD (Mothers Against Drunk Drivers),* and the lame advertising of beer manufacturers to "drink responsibly," society does not have effective programs to counteract this well-known problem. In addicts with millions of brain cells screaming for pleasure, there is little hope that "just saying no" is an effective deterrent (as observed in the Reagan Administration's failed drug policy).

Due to the element of *sexual perversity* inherent in serial killers, the "toxic" cocktail created by high testosterone levels and *ethanol* (the addictive chemistry that gets you drunk in beer, wine, and liquor) cannot be ignored as causative factors in serial homicide. FBI databases confirm that almost all *organized* serial killers use alcohol or other drugs during the commission of their crimes.

■ Id, Libido, & Sexual Innuendo

It is interesting that Freud championed the libido-driven, wish-fulfilling components of personality (or mind) as **id** impulses. If id could talk, maintained Freud, it would say: "I want it NOW!" This shows the **hedonistic** qualities of the metaphorical id and lack of restraint, not only in conscious experiences but also unconsciously, even as id threatens to disrupt sleep. (Today, we know that testosterone, dopamine (DA), Phenylethylamine (PEA), and norepinephrine (NE) contribute in varying degrees to the feeling of hedonism, and therefore, chemically compose id.)

Parenthetically, to Freud, dreams preserved sleep by disguising libido (or sex drive)—the driving force beyond sexual fantasies—with more socially acceptable symbols, such as cars, cigars, umbrellas, and boxes. In his first of many psychological *faux pas,* Freud provided his distracters plenty of ammunition to discredit his theories. Any elongated object in dreams, Freud theorized, was symbolic of a penis; any cavernous space should be interpreted as vaginal. Interestingly, distracters of Freud insist "sometimes a cigar is just a cigar," dispelling Freud's insistence that all dreams must have symbolic components of *sexual innuendo.* Apparently, if Freud were alive today he would not be surprised to see the number of sexualized crimes since a central point of his **conflict theory** was man's inability to control id—the original "system" of personality lying behind the **pleasure principle** and libido.

We mention this aspect of Freud's theory to show serial predators can be understood as "id-driven" sexual deviants, according to Freudian theory. Regarding his focus on conflict and sexuality, Freud might send a message from the grave to modern criminal investigators: "I told you so."

■ "Cooling Off"

In serial crimes, a "cooling off" period occurs between murders. From FBI research, during "cooling off" periods, serial predators often remained jazzed by viewing pornography; they may revisit or re-live crimes by visiting crime scenes or cemeteries, or by caressing their crime scene "trophies," or obsess over their macabre "photo gallery" of crime scene photographs. In addition, serial homicides of the *organized* variety show attention to detail, planning, and execution over and above that observed in a spree, mass murder, or disorganized topologies.

According to the Jacobs (2003) and his criminal profiling students, many of whom have taken introduction to psychology, the *organized serial killer* appears to have the following psychological proclivities. The *organized serial killer* . . .

1. Is more *obsessive-compulsive* than the disordered serial killer due to planning, detailing, and prolonging every detail of the crime as long as possible.
2. Relies on more *socially approved personas* than the disordered serial killer, who often appears unkempt (depicted as a "drifter" and/or a "dirty old man" stereotype).
3. Appears more of an *extrovert*—using "people skills" rather than the detached *introverted* loner.
4. Follows an **internal locus of control** (ILOC) rather than an external one. The ILOC-directed killer is more confident that he can get away with anything he plans through hard work, focus, and strategy. He has a "gift of gab"—he thinks he can talk his way out of any situation and often does. He feels intellectually superior to the authorities pursuing him.

■ Premenstrual Syndrome

For some females, a chemical condition **PMS (premenstrual syndrome)**, represents the darker, undesirable part of being a woman. During this part of her monthly cycle, women commonly suffer from a variety of discomforting symptoms such as headaches, fatigue, lethargy, tension, insomnia, and general irritability. For some women, PMS can initiate *uncontrollable wrath and acts of violence.* Premenstrual syndrome has been associated with crimes such as vandalism, aggravated assault, and even murder. According to research, some women during PMS are capable of anything, including crime. According to some medical researchers: "The most common psychological symptoms include depression, irritability, lethargy . . . however, these feelings can lead to criminal behavior."

According to David A. Gershaw Ph.D., PMS can have far-reaching consequences. He gives an example of two women in England whose murder sentences were reduced because they were under the stress from PMS. Researchers found that pre-menstrual women are more prone to accidents and injuries, being admitted to a mental hospital, or calling in sick to work. The implications are clear. A female who has a preexisting anger management issue may be more likely to commit a violent crime during PMS. According to Scutt (1982), two out of every ten women have "symptoms of sufficient severity every month to interfere with their ability to function normally." As previously mentioned regarding ADD or ADHD, no serious researcher is prepared to suggest that one single root causer—PMS—causes females to become killers.

The following is a survey form duplicated from an Internet site used to determine whether or not a woman has severe enough symptoms of PMS to cause her real emotional problems. Respondents complete the form by answering "yes" or "no."

1. Do you display aggressive behavior toward your partner and children?
2. Does depression, irritability, lethargy, or all of the above affect your daily activities?
3. Which affects you the most: depression, irritability, lethargy, or all of the above?
4. When are your symptoms the most severe: four days before menstruation, or four days after, or both?
5. Do you encounter a lot of stress?
6. Do you feel guilty when you are pre-menstruating?
7. Do you consume an alcoholic beverage?

Apparently, respondents who answer "yes" to the majority of the questions are the most at risk.

■ Behavioral Paradigm: Learning Amid Dysfunction

Spawned by the rise and heyday of behaviorism in the 1920s–1950s in North American psychology, **aberrant** behavior (as well as criminal behavior) was observed as nothing more than "conditioned" or learned behavior. Learning occurs by either *pairing two events together* (classical conditioning) or by reinforcing, punishing, removing, or ignoring behavior through *behavioral consequences* (operant conditioning). Behaviorists argue that both learning paradigms—classical and operant conditioning—produce behavior that is functional, dysfunctional, or criminal. So-called "soft" behaviorists (those who study cognition in addition to behavior) add **social modeling** and **cognitive mapping**.

According to operant conditioning principles (BF Skinner and his "school" of behaviorism), *emitted behavior* is shaped and maintained by consequences. **Emitted behavior** is defined as behavior not tied to any specific stimulus, which behaviorists' contend accounts for most human behavior. Hence, dysfunctional (and criminal) behavior comes from reinforced behavior in dysfunctional milieus by incompetent and/or absent parenting, and antisocial (toxic) parenting.

Behaviorists recognize the following behavioral consequences to represent feedback from emitted behavior due to conditioning "**operants**"—any behavior capable of being reinforced.

1. Positive reinforcement (behavior reinforced by *positive consequences* such as smiles, attention, love, or money),
2. Negative reinforcement (any behavior used *to remove* negative consequences or annoying behavior),
3. Ignoring (withholding attention), and
4. Punishment (physical or corporal such as hitting or spanking that discourages behavior).

Normally, most individuals tend to repeat behaviors that are positively reinforced. Attention and smiles encourage interpersonal relationships, while frowns and looks of displeasure are negative reinforcers—feedback that prompts individuals to remove the behavior that produced the negative feedback. Behavior that is ignored removes the powerful stimulus of attention. Theoretically, a person who is ignored will eventually give up due to lack of attention. Finally, punishment refers to the corporal variety—spanking or hitting another person to associate pain as a consequence of undesirable behavior.

According to *learning theory,* perhaps the "becoming" psychopath has been largely ignored and/or routinely punished by incompetent or hateful parenting to the point that important brain areas (i.e. limbic system, prefrontal lobes, or cerebellum) have failed to develop a normal array of synaptic connections. Raised in dysfunctional and/or abusive milieus, young children have minimal experience with positive reinforcement from nourishing, attentive, and loving parents. Due to emotional scarcity, the brain can fail to "wire" itself normally.

Incarcerated serial killers report that parents doled out harsh and/or inconsistent punishment and ignored them (many serial killers felt they were boarders in their own homes) producing the early "conditioning" of psychopathy.

As behavioral underpinnings of criminality from a behavioral perspective, a cursory overview of classical and operant conditioning follows:

■ S→R Psychology: Classical Conditioned Responses

In classical conditioning (or **S→R psychology**), learning is synonymous with "conditioning" so that new behavior is conditioned by associating two stimuli together. The unconditioned stimulus—the UCS—is naturally stimulating (hence "unconditioned). By paring a neutral stimulus with the UCS, new learning occurs. In the famous experiment in classical conditioning, Pavlov's dogs salivated to the bell (CS) because the bell was paired with food (UCS). By the same process, sexualized predators are only erotically "jazzed" to a specific victim (CS) because of paring him/her with violent pornography or other eroticized material (UCS) compulsively viewed in pornographic movies.

◼ Fetishism

A **fetish**, for example, is learned in the same way Pavlov's dog salivated to the bell. A conditioned stimulus occurs by associating an object (such as hosiery—the CS) with sexual fantasy from viewing erotic videos, which naturally causes a person to become sexually aroused (UCS). Because serial perpetrators are *sexual deviates,* fetish burglaries of women's panties, bras, or other articles of intimate apparel tintilate at first, then escalate into more serious offenses such as rape or murder. Yet, more serious crimes are predictable as the serial predator "demands" more physical "connection" to a real victim than an earlier fetish produced.

According to classical conditioning and the well-established **law of association** in a crime of retribution, for example, due to earlier conditioning—pairing an emotionally unpleasant event with a given person—a victim is targeted. The bad experience "festers" in the perpetrator's mind over time producing negative thinking and the desire to retaliate and settle the score. Bad feelings become intertwined and associated with the targeted person (as a conditioned stimulus) to the point that just seeing the person (CS) causes the person to feel anger and hostility. Never having learned effective coping skills, restraint, or less harmful ways to vent anger, the person starts to obsess and be consumed with anger and eventually "loses it" and "acts out" harming the targeted person.

In all sexualized crimes, pairing hardcore, violent sex to females (or to a specific typology, such as a female with blonde hair, long legs, or big breasts), for example, the female, or parts of her body, become the CS—the target. The implication to the psychopath is that all females enjoy being sexualized in this way. Why not? This is how females are portrayed—as victims, who are rarely empowered in "porn" films. Again, pornography is the unconditioned stimulus (UCS) paired to the chosen female victim (in the organized offender) who becomes the conditioned stimulus (CS). Both the unconditioned response (UCR) and the conditioned response (CR) are the same—*erotic feeling* leading in most cases to orgasm.

As a result of pairing, any number or variety of females he encounters in everyday life are candidates for CSs. The lonely, sexual psychopath is excited (and perhaps already addicted) to overpowering a female and "giving her what she deserves" just like the deviant sex he views everyday in his "porn" collection.

Psychopaths have never learned socially appropriate ways to interact with others or vent anger through jogging, working out, or slugging a punching bag. Mostly likely, *he has never had consensual sex.* Organized serial killers drive though neighborhoods or specific areas such as parks or around convenience stores in search of female victims who fit his deviant fantasies.

◼ Operant Conditioning Paradigm

In operant conditioning, deviant behavior is reinforced with *behavioral consequences* by loveless and abusive parents—rightly called antisocial parenting. For healthy development, children require predictable milieus, a context not found in dysfunctional homes. Severely dysfunctional parenting produces anger and frustration leading to deviant behavior in their stressed-out children. Predictably, unhappy and angry children seek outlets for their displeasure, which often leads to behavioral **chaining**, where perverted behavior is *linked together,* leading to more serious breaches of conduct. As an example, cruelty to animals and petty crimes escalate into major ones, seemingly overnight. Teenagers who have a history of antisocial parenting evidenced by repressed anger and/or depression, feel abandoned, lonely, and "different" and are on a collision course with psychopathy.

Recently, with three shots from a high-powered hunting rifle, a seventeen-year old male student, days from graduating from high school, killed a rival peer on the school parking lot. He sought affection, as did the victim, a former boyfriend of the same girlfriend. Weeks earlier, he had written graphic descriptions of how the bullets would puncture his rival's skin and produce a rapid flow of blood. In behavioral terms, the victim became the conditioned CS—"standing for" hurt feelings experienced by the revenge-seeking killer.

◼ The Law of Effect

In operant conditioning, the "becoming" psychopath has received a lifetime of dysfunctional behavioral feedback from parents, peers, and others. (The word "operant" comes from B. F. Skinner's brand of **radical behaviorism** describing how humans and animals "operate" on their environments and how feedback shapes and maintains behavior without need of analyzing cognition.)

Earlier, Edward Thorndike of Columbia University discovered "satisfiers" and "annoyers" in the behavior of cats trying to escape a puzzle box. Behavior that led to escape to a food dish were repeated over and again in a predictable fashion (satisfiers) leading Thorndike to formulate his famous **Law of Effect**, stating behavior followed by positive consequences is strengthened while behavior followed by "annoyers" was weakened. The cats quickly learned where the "payoff," or rather the means to the payoff, was located—around the triggering mechanism of the latch. In a few trials, the cats ran directly to the latch as a means of escape to the food dish. Is human behavior so different?

Perversity of the Law of Effect

A perversity of the Law of Effect occurs when a serial killer's rapacious behavior produces "positive" consequences—fulfilling (somewhat) his deviant fantasies—by engaging in lust, mutilation, and ultimately macabre behavior. What is the emotional "payoff" necessary in the Law of Effect that controls behavior so predictably? The emotional "payoff" to the serial predator is always found in his *signature*—the desire to control, dominate, manipulate, and ultimately to derive sexual gratification through sexual exploitation. Signature is his *fait accompli* of serial killing.

Antisocial parenting reinforces deviant behavior in children in part by being such poor role models—parents who are alcoholics, abusers, molesters, and emotionally paralyzed **enablers**—allowing children to continue being dysfunctional without appropriate consequence. A good example of enabling occurred with the parents of Jeffrey Dahmer who failed to intercede with his obsession of autopsying road kill. How could his parents have not known his **nefarious** ritual? Ignoring Dahmer's road kill ritual allowed his dysfunctional behavior to progress. As more perverted thinking occurred, Dahmer eventually committed his first murder. Reinforcing deviant behavioral expectations by modeling it, and by ignoring it, encourages the behavior to continue.

Regardless, from both classical and operant perspectives, children become psychopathic because of *learned behavior* in severely pathological family and peer milieus. We doubt a "sexual psychopathy gene" will be discovered in follow up studies to the *Human Genome Project*. In addition, the following contribute to antisocial behavior:

1. Maladaptive or ineffective coping skills and lack of restraint learned from incompetent, absent, hateful, and antisocial parenting,
2. Anger and frustration from lack of observed nurturing/attention, and love,
3. Obsession with violent sexual fantasies, where control and manipulation (compulsion) replace "give-and-take" of normal relationships. A steady diet of hardcore pornography and other forms of eroticized violence in mass media or on the Internet contribute, as well as obsession with violent and sexually exploitative video games, which further exacerbates psychopathy.

■ "Soft Behaviorism"

The "soft" behaviorist perspective (in the tradition of cognitive-behaviorist Albert Bandura, Edward Tolman, and others) proposes the development of deviant cognitive maps of thinking, fueling sexualized fantasy that leads to criminal behavior. Loveless antisocial parenting provides social modeling of deviant behavior in a scenario of "monkey see-monkey do."

Interestingly, the social-cognitive perspective to learning, being less tied to strict empirical controls of laboratory settings, had nothing to do with psychology "losing its mind" to the strict behavioral theories of Watson and Skinner.

FBI agents and co-founders modern criminal profiling, Robert Ressler and John Douglas used exclusively the introspective "self-report" in gaining insight into criminal behavior from incarceration interviews. Can incarcerated criminals be believed? Apparently yes, especially when subsequent behavior from criminals accused of similar crimes shows similar behavioral patterns. Behavioral patterns set up contingencies and probabilities that forecast predictable behavior. Results and experience ultimately approve or disapprove the introspective approach of gathering information. (The introspective approach is precisely how Freud developed his theory and treatment of hysteria.)

Behavioral psychology, (learning theory), is committed to *learning paradigms*. The cornerstone of behavior is that personality is learned and is manifested in behavior. To behaviorists, sexual deviance is a learned behavior exemplified in the 1950s with "The Lonely Hearts Killer" Harvey Glatman.

PREDATOR PROFILE (3-1)

Harvey Murray Glatman
"The Lonely Hearts Killer"

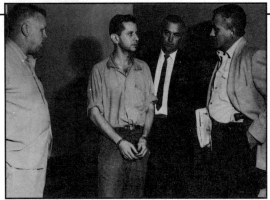

©Bettmann/CORBIS

Crime Span:

August 1957 to October 1958

Physical Description:

Harvey Glatman was a white male, 140 lbs. He had large "dumbo" ears and visible pock-marks from acne on his face. He had squinty eyes and messy hair. On occasion, he wore horn-rim glasses.

As a child, Harvey Glatman was perceived to be "a little strange" by his own parents. At the age of four, he was caught in a sadomasochistic act, consisting of a string tied around his penis with the loose end in a drawer. He leaned back against the string, causing pain. He enjoyed self-punishment. The string proved to a prescient metaphor of things to come; the string became a rope he used around his neck in an obsession with *autoerotic asphyxia* as an adolescent. Glatman tied a rope around his neck and looped the free end over a rafter. He then yanked the rope with one hand and masturbated with the other. He envisioned the ropes as extensions of his arms. As a serial killer, he used rope on his victims to bind them so he could control and manipulate them.

In high school, Glatman committed a series of break-ins. Some were random, while others were carefully planned. The planned break-ins occurred after he followed an attractive girl to her home or apartment. He broke in her home and fondled her. He did not rape her. He was sentenced to a year in the Colorado State Prison in 1945 when he was just 17 years of age after being caught in a break-in.

Glatman was released from prison in July of 1946. He promptly moved to New York where he attempted several muggings with rape "in mind." He was apprehended and served nearly two more years of incarceration.

Psychiatrists diagnosed him "psychopathic personality-schizophrenic type," with "sexually perverted impulses." He learned how to trick the prison system by pretending to be a model prisoner. Upon his release, he headed for Los Angeles, California.

Victimology:

1. Judy Dull (August, 1957)

Glatman obtained her phone number from her agency. He identified himself as "Johnny Glenn." He lied to her saying he had seen her model before and wanted her to pose for the layout of a true crime magazine. Glatman picked up Dull and convinced her to go to his "studio," which, in reality, was his own apartment.

He tied her up, ostensibly, to photograph a bondage scene for the magazine. Once incapacitated, he pointed a gun at her, untied her, and ordered her to strip as he took pictures. Glatman then raped her several times. He transported her to the California desert where he killed her. He took pictures of the corpse.

2. Shirley Ann Bridgeford (March, 1958)

Shirley Ann Bridgeford joined the Patty Sullivan *Lonely Hearts Club* where she met "George Williams" (aka Harvey Glatman) and accepted a date with Williams. Glatman picked up Bridgeford for the "date" and drove her into the foothills of the Vallecito Mountains in California. He pointed a gun at her and forced her to strip. He took pictures of her and, subsequently, he killed her. He took more pictures of the corpse as he positioned her body.

3. Ruth Mercado (Angela Rojos) (July, 1958)

Glatman tricked the part-time stripper into thinking she was doing a photo shoot. Posing as a photographer, he entered her home where he raped her and then kidnapped her. Although she tried to put on a smile and go along with what she thought was a charade, he eventually strangled her with a rope. He dumped her body in the desert not far from the location of Bridgeford's body.

MO Features:

Glatman posed as a photographer and asked his victims to look "innocent" for the camera. He asked them to pose as if they were dead. Following the rape and murder of victims, he photographed the corpses, keeping the pictures as souvenirs. Glatman strangled all three victims with the same piece of rope.

Outcome:

After a failed attempt on the life of his last victim, Harvey Glatman was apprehended. After intense questioning, Glatman confessed to the murders. Also, he confessed to having a toolbox full of souvenirs. In a three-day trial, Glatman was convicted and sentenced to San Quentin were he died in the gas chamber in September of 1959. Glatman requested to be hanged as his death sentence (one last autoerotic event); nevertheless, he died from inhaling toxic gas.

Student Contributors:

Neil Tilly, Meghan Henn, and Valerie Warren, PA

◼ FBI's Investigative Paradigm— Criminal Profiling

Following physics (the most mathematical of all sciences) in the seventeenth and eighteenth centuries, and the rise of the natural sciences—biology and chemistry—in the nineteenth century, *empirical analysis* of behavior became the cultural *zeitgeist*. Spurred by **British empiricism** and **phenomenology**, and the German birth of Wundt's "lab psychology" in 1879, the importance of individual *experiences* contributing to unique aspects of personality came into focus. *Behavioral experiences* provide the segue from philosophy (with a focus on cognition) to psychology (with a focus on feeling). This transition occurred early in the twentieth century.

The language—terms, concepts, and methodology of psychology and psychiatry—became beacons of enlightenment to post-World War II North America. Those who resisted the florid language of the behavioral sciences often referred to its specialized lexica as psychobabble. But, **psychobabble**, especially of the Freudian variety (e.g. oedipal complex, repression) was *au courant* in the pop culture of the 1950s–1960s, as it remains today.

First, in the novels of Canon-Doyle, and later, during the Human Potential Movement of the early 1960s, a systematic attempt in law enforcement was underway to understand the criminal mind by *paying attention to his behavior*—to his psychology—at the crime scene and what it suggested about his personality. A few investigators were learning how this could elevate investigation to a new level by paying attention to a new investigative tool—assessing sexual psychopathy through criminal profiling.

◼ Teten & Mullany

Law enforcement professionals often bring personal methods of profiling gained through experience working in municipal law enforcement (such as police departments) when hired by the Federal Bureau of Investigation (FBI). One such individual, Howard Teten, once worked for a California police department, gained further insights and theory into the **etiology** of criminal behavior from attending the School of Criminology at the University of California. When he became a special agent of the FBI, he teamed with another agent, Pat Mullany, who taught abnormal psychology as a mandatory course for special agents of the FBI. Dating back to 1969 when Teten taught his first class of Applied Criminology, they launched what would become modern criminal profiling (with the contributions of Ressler, Douglas, and others).

Teten gained further insight into profiling when he consulted with Dr. James Brussel, a Greenwich Village psychiatrist, who solved the Mad Bomber case in New York in the mid-1950s.

By studying crime scene photographs and letters written by the bomber to local newspaper, Dr. Brussel pieced together *behavioral patterns,* including evidence of the bomber's **paranoia**. In Brussel's perspective, behavioral patterns suggest personality traits, the underlying psychological principle that continues today at the core of the FBI criminal profile.

At FBI headquarters, Teten and Mullany's merged their profiling methods with respective course material to hatch the *Applied Criminology* paradigm, the original system of profiling that has undergone numerous refinements beginning in the late 1970s.

▇ The "First Force"—From Behavioral Science to Investigative Support

The team of Teten and Mullany comprised the "first force" of FBI criminal-personality profilers (as profiling was referred to in the 1970s–1980s.) Upon his appointment to Behavioral Science, Special Agent John Douglas renamed the *Behavioral Science Unit* (BSU) the *Investigative Support Unit* (ISU), which is today part of the FBI's *National Center for the Analysis of Violent Crimes (NCAVC),* a major component of the *Critical Incident Response Group (CIRGE).*

How much bureaucracy has crept into the present system versus the original system of data gathering in compiling *known offender characteristics* is anyone's guess. (Interestingly, the impetus behind Douglas dropping the "Behavioral Science" name came from the initials "BS," suggesting fellow agents and others held a **pejorative** view of the fledging unit.) Regardless, the unit consisted of agents with academic training in:

1. Abnormal psychology (psychopathology),
2. Behavioral psychology (behaviorism),
3. Forensic science (evidence headed to the courtroom), and
4. Additional psychological perspectives gained from professionals in mental health agencies.

The *Investigative Support Unit (ISU)* provides adjunct training to a diverse group of professionals such as lawyers, psychologists, and detectives from all over the world.

Alluded to in Chapter One, the ISU has accumulated an immense database regarding known offender behavior, relative to the following perpetrator characteristics. This database has obvious parallels to a clinical document, the psychosocial history; perpetrator characteristics include:

1. General background (family, work, and individual history)
2. Family dynamics
3. Current behavioral tendencies
4. Psychological characteristics

Regardless of how profiling strategies became part of a special agents training, the FBI's *Behavioral Science Unit (BSU),* through a succession of special agents, is given credit for initiating and developing criminal profiling. But as we have shown, variations on the theme of profiling existed long before that time in municipal law enforcement, autopsies, and in clinical psychiatry with assessment protocol.

In today's *zeitgeist,* "forensics" is a hot topic. Court TV programs routinely show how physical evidence—marks, wounds, tissue analysis, and offender "graffiti" are analyzed through the expertise and speculative logic of "celebrity" forensic pathologists, notably Dr. Henry Lee and Dr. Michael

Baden. Truly, pathologists need just a spot of blood, or one case, a single tooth to "create" a whole person.

■ FBI Profiling Methods

The FBI's method of profiling, spawned a half-century ago, favors *statistical data basing*. This generates *inductive* inferences by comparing current offender behavior with prior offender behavior, victimology, and crime scene data. Again, this approach is termed "inductive" and "empirical" due to linking the present to the past (cause and effect) in a systematized, objective fashion, much like the DSM documents psychological disorders observed over years of clinical experience. What modern day profilers learn about present crimes is used to "modernize" serial offender protocols.

According to criminal profiling analysts Cantor and Turvey, the real problem in all profiling perspectives is formidable: most investigators have received *inadequate training in analyzing crime scene data*—the single most important part of the profiling document. As a result, they often embark upon any one of the more *subjective* profiling perspectives. For criminal investigators who are weak in analyzing crime scene evidence, they, by necessity, turn to the FBI databases to fill in the gaps.

John Douglas (*Anatomy of Motive, Journey into Darkness*) suggests the profiling process is a seven step evaluative process. Profilers evaluate:

1. The criminal act (actus reus). Profilers study *modus operandi* (MO)—the method of operation (small steps) taken as the crime materializes at the crime scene, as well as the emotional "signature"—behavior thrills that compel him to kill again.
2. Specifics of the crime scene.
3. Victimology (victim characteristics and why he or she was chosen).
4. Preliminary police reports.
5. Medical examiner's autopsy report.
6. Profiles specific offender characteristics.
7. Investigative procedures suggested by the profile.

General Aphorisms of Profiling

Once a profiler starts to compile *general biographical* information that eventually targets an UNSUB, a series of unsolved offenses, such as fires, rapes, or stalking, may be linked to the same perpetrator. It is imperative to start with the suspect's *history of early crimes* in an effort to target the vicinity of his residence. In this instance of speculative logic, the profiler observes that serial killers often start with lesser offenses in his own back yard, his comfort zone. At first, he operates like a trapdoor spider prowling around places of great familiarity, situated close to where he lives and works. He comes out in a brief bust of criminal activity and recedes into his "trapdoor." As he gains more confidence and experience, his activity radius usually expands, making his geographical point of origin more difficult to specify.

Serial killers usually select a *certain type of victim* possessing traits that are sexually appealing to him (facial features, color/style of hair, body type, breast size, type of dress, etc). **Idiosyncratic** focus best describes the selection of the perpetrator's choice of victims. As we have seen, at the root of serial murder lies the ever-present sexual psychopathy, crimes committed by a sexual deviant with a mind neurologically damaged beyond repair.

■ Crime Scene Analysis

In 1978, FBI special agents, Robert Ressler and John Douglas modified the Teten-Mullany *Applied Criminology Model* of serial killers into the *Organized/Disorganized Model.* This model remains influential today. From 1979–1983, FBI agents hatched the *Criminal Personality Research Project,* the dream and literary "child" of FBI special agent Robert Ressler. The undertaking was truly a landmark for the FBI, who at the time (ironically) showed limited interest in what motivated murderers, rapists, and child molesters. (Incidentally, all of the offenses are not against federal law.) The study took dead aim at the *psychological and behavioral characteristics* of violent criminals related to backgrounds, specific crimes, crime scenes, and victimology.

Special agents of the FBI obtained this information first-hand by entering correctional facilities initially before or after "road schools" where agents taught FBI techniques to local law enforcement agencies. Talking with offenders *vis a vis* and augmenting personal interviews by homework, poring though stacks of forensic evidence—court transcripts, psychiatric assessments, and police reports—the exhaustive study resulted in the creation of a list of crime scene protocols known as *Crime Scene Analysis (CSA).*

The current dichotomy of *organized versus disorganized model* follows the presentation of the six steps of the CSA paradigm; which are:

1. *Profiling Inputs.* The initial stage of CSA refers to evidence gathering. All *crime scene materials* gathered at the crime scene, such as photographs of the crime scene and/or victim. Evidence such as comprehensive background information on the victim, autopsy reports, and forensic information relative to the "psychological autopsy" of the crime scene—postulating what occurred before, during, and after the crime. Profiling Inputs serve as the foundation of the CSA. Any errors and/or miscalculations in this *evidence gathering* stage can lead investigators in wrong directions.

2. *Decision Process Models.* *Logistics* is the best word to describe the second stage of CSA. What must emerge from this stage is a *logical* and *coherent pattern,* the emerging picture of the perpetrator suggested by the crime scene, such as whether or not a serial perpetrator was responsible, or if the evidence points to a single instance of a crime (the offender's one and only crime).

3. *Crime Assessment. Crime reconstruction* best describes the third stage. What are the sequence of events and behavioral characteristics of victim and offender? What "role" did the victim play? What "role" did the

offender play? Analyzing this stage allows investigators to gradually piece together the emerging criminal profile.

4. *Criminal Profile.* The actual profile starts to take place with the fourth protocol with background data, behavioral characteristics, and physical description of the perpetrator. If apprehended, this stage provides suggestions of the most effective ways to *interview* the offender based on personality type. *Identification and apprehension* of the offender is the goal of this stage.

5. *Investigation.* This is the *application phase* where law enforcement agencies are provided with the actual profile to aid in the apprehension of the perpetrator. New information modifies the original profile, sometimes on a day-to-day basis.

6. *Apprehension.* Crosschecking the profile with the apprehended offender is the last stage of CSA. This stage has built-in difficulties in the event the offender is never caught, or the offender is arrested on another charge, or the offender ceases criminal activity.

◼ Turf Wars

Due to simple logistics and familiarity with a given region and its citizens, local law enforcement agencies have long believed their own efforts of criminal apprehension are superior to FBI involvement. Yet, the FBI model remains a widely sought system of criminal apprehension worldwide as observed in the bureau's *Fellowship Program,* where law enforcement personnel from around the world travel to Quantico, Virginia to learn the idiosyncracies of profiling and *Crime Scene Analysis.*

◼ Organized/Disorganized Offender Dichotomy

The following taxonomy represents behavioral characteristics of violent crime offenders relative to the *Organized Offender* characteristics.

The Organized Offender

The *organized serial killer* is suggested by the following behavioral characteristics:

1. Average to above average intelligence
2. Socially competent
3. Skilled work preferred
4. Sexually competent
5. High birth order status
6. Father's work stable
7. Inconsistent childhood discipline

8. Controlled mood during crime
9. Use of alcohol during crime
10. Precipitating situational stress
11. Living with partner
12. Mobility with car in good condition
13. Follows crime in news media
14. May change jobs or leave town

SOURCE: *Whoever Fights Monsters* (Ressler 1992).

The Disorganized Offender

The *disorganized serial killer* is suggested by the following behavioral characteristics:

1. Below average intelligence
2. Socially inadequate
3. Unskilled worker
4. Sexually incompetent
5. Low birth order status
6. Father's work unstable
7. Harsh discipline as a child
8. Anxious mood during crime
9. Minimal use of alcohol
10. Minimal situational stress
11. Living alone
12. Lives/works near the crime scene
13. Minimal interest in news media
14 Significant behavior change (ex. Drug/alcohol abuse)

SOURCE: *Whoever Fights Monsters* (Ressler 1992).

■ Organized Predator Poster Boy: Ted Bundy

The "poster-boy" predator for the *organized offender* is the serial killer Theodore "Ted" Bundy. It is instructive to apply his personal vita in the following delineation of organized versus disorganized offenders.

In terms of IQ (Intelligence Quotient), the organized offender is almost always average to above average in intelligence (Bundy was in law school at the time of his offenses and possessed a "gift of gab" along with above average academic skills). In contrast, the disorganized offender is usually below average in intelligence and may not have a high school diploma or a GED.

The organized offender is *socially component* and sophisticated, meaning he has a grasp on the way society "works" and possesses the requisite interpersonal skills to maintain at least a persona of normal social relationships. Bundy made friends easily and possessed strong manipulative skills. The judge who presided over his murder trial berated Bundy for his offenses (paraphrased) "I would have liked to hear you argue in court someday . . . you would have been a good lawyer . . . but you chose the wrong path." The organized offender is proficient at acquiring and keeping skilled jobs, as was the case with the offender's father. Bundy was adopted into a home with a stepfather who had a stable work record.

The disorganized offer is socially incompetent, displaying socially inadequate behavior such as disturbed or nonexistent social relationships and is a "job-hopper," an unskilled laborer following in the footsteps of his father's spotty work history.

The organized offender often has success in sexual relationships with girlfriends, wives, or ex-wives. Bundy had girlfriends and even married one of his admirers who witnessed the trial. While in prison, conjugal visits by his wife produced a daughter.

The disorganized offender is sexually incompetent. Interviewed on death row, disorganized offenders report never having experienced a mutually satisfying sexual relationship with another. The disorganized offender bases sex on control, domination, degradation, and/or abuse.

A history of inconsistent discipline characterizes the organized offender's childhood. Researchers have documented this fact in Bundy's parent-child relationship. On the other hand, harsh discipline characterizes the disorganized offender's history of discipline.

During the commission of the crime, the mood of the organized offender is somewhat stable, enhanced with the abuse of alcohol. Bundy was intoxicated during the commission of his crimes. The disorganized offender's mood is anxious with minimal use of alcohol during the commission of the crime.

There exists a precipitating stressor or "trigger" to the crime for organized offenders (having to leave law school due to finances was the "trigger" in Bundy's case), while minimal situational stressors exist in the behavior of disorganized offenders.

Organized offenders live with a partner (a wife or girlfriend), while disorganized offenders live alone. Due to a total lack of transportation or fear of mechanical breakdown, the disorganized offender lives close to the crime scene, while the organized offender displays a wider range of mobility with dependable transportation. Bundy drove a VW beetle in good repair.

The disorganized offender displays minimal interest in the media coverage. The organized offender follows news coverage avidly (true in Bundy's case). After the crime, the organized offender may leave town or change jobs. Bundy left town, eventually moving state to state. In contrast, while the disorganized offender never strays from home, his behavior changes radically as observed in increased drug and/or alcohol abuse.

◼ Behavior Reflects Personality

As introduced in Chapter One, profiling (at least from the perspective of the FBI paradigm), is committed to the behavioral aphorism: *behavior reflects personality*. Profilers expect sexual psychopaths to display behavior and personality characteristics denoting perverted, sexualized behavior evident at the crime scene with a distinctive signature.

Police departments, as well as the FBI, use profiling to refine their suspect list with general biographical information, often targeting perpetrators with uncanny accuracy. Additionally, the expression "to go proactive" means lending enough information to news reports to allow the general public to become a "partner" in solving the crime. A million or more sets of eyes are better than one.

The following eclectic psychological principles will be recognizable to psychology students from divergent perspectives within general psychology. Do they further elucidate the mind of sexual psychopaths? Here's a list of psychological issues that touch upon post-adolescent development of serial killers:

■ Intimacy versus Isolation

Normal couples explore sexuality on the way to intimacy. *Intimacy is far from just the physical act of sex.* Intimacy involves nurturing, care, trust, and "being there" through all the ups and downs inherent in modern relationships. Intimacy is paying attention to the smallest details of love and sharing, and providing financial and emotional support. Above all, intimacy is love, caring, and protection of mate and family.

Many developmental psychologists believe the development of intimacy to be the most critical of all Eriksonian stages of psychosocial development. When the crisis of intimacy has been experienced and "internalized," couples can emotionally nourish each other and their children.

"Rootedness" within intimacy may be the single most important "glue" to long-lasting relationships. On the other hand, the sexual psychopath feels disconnected and lonely. In the place of normalcy, deviant behavior exerts devastating results. A lover's kiss and intimate touch is replaced by the predator's **rapacious** and deadly "embrace" of death. Due to feeling depersonalized through incompetent parenting, the psychopath feels isolation in every part of his being. His anger is close to rage and only lacks a "trigger" to set him off.

We purpose that irreversible neurological harm has already been done (perhaps the most devastating before 2 years of age, and then additionally up to ten-years-of-age) as psychopathy renders the perpetrator incapable of intimacy through *reciprocity*. Feeling lonely and isolated in critical developmental stages, he often "acts out" inappropriately. He may sit alone and fantasize about the polar opposites of sexual intimacy, caring, and love, that is, rape, control, and murder.

As we will soon discover in Chapter Four, Erik Erikson's developmental stage occurring in the age group most populated by serial killers (ages 20s to early 40s) is the *crisis of intimacy versus isolation* providing-compelling evidence of the effects of persistent antisocial parenting from birth to late adolescence.

The emotional crises of each antecedent stage were met with frustration, lack of emotional bonding, and absence of tender emotions expected from nurturing. As we will see, psychopathy results from severe emotional scarcity and abuse resulting in irreversible neurological damage. This occurred due to the scarcity of positive feelings. At every developmental stage, antisocial parents failed their children.

■ Cognitive Neuroscience—Focus

It is a well-established principle of **cognitive psychology** and a closely related discipline **cognitive neuroscience** that focus controls the direction and energy of one's life. The **aphorism**—"thinking wags the tail of behavior"—best captures the central influence of focus. Serial killers are obsessively focused on total *domination* of victims, accomplished through manipulation, deception, and/or catching victims "off guard." To prolong the attack, during the assault, the perpetrator may use a **garrote** to slowly strangle the victim. When the victim passes out, the perpetrator loosens the noose. As she slowly recovers, he continues his assault. When she recovers enough oxygen to resist, he tightens the noose again. This is repeated many times during the assault to prolong the perpetrators murderous fantasies. Eventually the victim dies.

Addiction to pornography in all its forms—violent crime scene magazines, and other graphic illustrations of sexualized violence—fuel the scary inner world of killers. When the killer is apprehended, authorities expect to find physical evidence of his obsession—magazines, videotapes, and sexually deviant Web sites reflecting his perverted cognitive focus.

Neuropsychology, psychology at the tissue level, and cognitive neuroscience contend that sexual psychopaths' time, energy, and focus are captured by a sexually perverse addiction, an addiction, perhaps ironically, to their own brain chemistry.

■ Dual Diagnosis

To be more accurate, serial killers should require an additional psychiatric label known as **dual diagnosis**, meaning some form of chemical dependency (of one or more drugs) exacerbates one or more major personality disorders. Even when his drug of choice is found, one fact must be addressed. Serial killers are addicted to the "thrilling high" associated with sexual tension and release, the same way brain chemistry "rewards" sexual behavior with pleasurable brain chemistry. Drugs can be used to lessen inhibition, prolong pleasurable feelings, or simply to *self-medicate* his "brutal urge" to continue rapacious crime.

Almost all serial killers have had their share of abuse, depravity, and/or emotional scarcity from antisocial parenting during early developmental stages. Dysfunctional parenting, or in some instances, a complete lack of parental involvement, leaves deep emotional scars. Never having achieved much, if anything worthwhile, young psychopaths are portrayed by criminologists as seething with revenge for those individuals perceived responsible. (Jeffrey Dahmer blamed his pent-up rage on the emotional distance of his father as well as "demons.")

Revenge is defined as pent-up emotion that is consciously experienced as *unsettling feelings*—perhaps a mixture of anger, rage, depression, and/or anxiety; it's highly subjective and idiosyncratic to the individual.

Macabre thoughts exacerbate the addictive "high" of neurochemistry in the pleasure pathways of the brain, setting up the *fait accompli* of sexualized murder—complete domination, control, and sexual experimentation followed by murder. Profilers discovered that many killers revisit crime scenes, or the shallow graves where they bury victims, in an effort to relive the experience "just one more time," largely through masturbation or necrophilia.

■ Personality Disorder NOS

Rather than the traditional antisocial personality disorder, a diagnosis of **personality disorder NOS, or PD NOS** (NOS means "not otherwise specified") is a more precise diagnosis for serial killers. A **PD NOS** means a more accurate diagnosis might include other features of personality disorders such as **narcissistic personality disorder** (or **borderline personality disorder**); features of one or both may occur in conjunction with the antisocial personality disorder.

Regardless, illicit drugs enhance a killer's primary addiction—*his own brain chemistry*. This effect can be compared to lovers' heightened pleasure as "energy" from foreplay, prolonging it during sex, and feeling "spent" in the aftermath.

Jungian **archetypes** observed in normal personality extend into the devi-ant personality of psychopaths with two recognizable characteristics: *Extraversion versus Introversion.*

A category of serial predators (especially those designated as *disorganized* offenders or those marked by a profound mental illness) kill close to home; in contrast, serial killers, designated as *organized* offenders with less mental anomalies, prefer to travel farther from home or constantly move about the country. Due to the pioneering work of Carl Jung, the archetypes of *extraversion* and *introversion* partially explain both the emotional and physical maneuverability of serial killers. Most likely, the organized offender variety is an affable **extravert**—a "people person" with accomplished social skills—a talker and social mixer, while the disorganized variety is a territorial **introvert**—a shy, brooding loner.

Like non-criminal counterparts, non-criminal extraverts need people to jazz their inner world, which researchers describe as "low gainers." The **reticular activation system (RAS)** of the brain "sets" stimulation levels for extraverts too low, meaning their internal dialogue is far too "quiet"; hence, they are driven to seek out other people and social opportunities to help stimulate their boring inner world. The organized serial killer—perhaps the extravert—seeks victims to rape and kill in an effort to fill the hole in his vacant inner world.

On the other hand, the non-criminal introvert has a "high gain" setting from the RAS, meaning he has plenty of "noise" and activity from his internal dialogue of ideas and thoughts. Therefore, he is practically a home-

Holmes' "Four Type" Paradigm

In an alternative paradigm, a criminologist from the University of Louisville, Ronald Holmes, proposes *four types of serial offenders:*

1. *The Visionary Type.* Hearing voices or seeing visions drives the visionary type to serial homicide where voices/visions command him to kill others. The visionary type is often **psychotic**. A recent movie, *Frailty,* depicted the visionary type of serial killer.

2. *The Mission-Oriented Type.* This type kills a specific group of people who he believes are unworthy to live and the world will be much better off without them "infesting" it. He is not psychotic and often viewed by acquaintances as a model citizen.

3. *The Hedonistic Type.* The "thrill-killer" who is jazzed sexually by the act of domination and degradation. He may linger for long periods of time at the crime scene performing acts of **necrophilia** on his victims.

4. *The Power-Oriented Type.* Killer who enjoys controlling and dominating victims though vocalizations and/or behavior.

 sexual psychopath

Sexual psychopathy seems most evident in Holmes' *hedonistic* and *power-oriented types*.

body who is territorial with his time and energy. He does not need people to stimulate him like the extravert who craves the nightlife and partying to make up for the "low gain" setting of the RAS.

Ted Bundy-types represent the organized, extraverted serial killer, while the Edmund Kemper-types represent the disorganized, introverted type.

◼ Psychological Determinism

Determinism states that **antecedent** events (especially in childhood) set up a "menu of selection" for present behavioral "choices." In determinism, the so-called "decisions" we make are not really based on capricious free will; "decisions" are very limited due to the narrow menu reflecting the only "choices" we could have made, given our limited "menu." In determinism, capricious free will is a complete illusion, or a fiction based upon ignorance of the power of antecedent experiences.

Ironically, both Freud and the behaviorists (especially Watson and Skinner) agreed with determinism as the ultimate "blueprint" for current and future behavior. The "red flags" of psychopathic behavior observed in the childhoods of Dahmer and Bundy, for example, set up limited menus of "choices." In this perspective, they did not "decide" in the coolness of thought to become serial killers in the sense of making a *conscious choice to murder* in the "coolness" of reason. Profilers have discovered that, in fact, some serial killers *panic when the victim offers resistance so they kill the victim to keep her quiet.*

The strong, sexualized content of the serial killer's deviant thinking produces persistent and compelling sexual fantasies, leaving but one "choice" on the "menu"—acting out in order to experience the equivalent of a mental "ejaculation"—a rush of pleasurable neurochemistry.

The key is how serial killers *feel* as they search for victims and fantasize the attack. Deviant thinking drives *feelings* set in motion by neurochemicals and hormonals, leading to addiction. This confluence of emotional events eventually "wags the tail of behavior."

◼ General Forensic Evidence

Elements that are necessary to produce the most accurate profile for use by law enforcement or for the courtroom are:

1. *Objectivity.* One of the elements of science, *objectivity* is absolutely necessary in generating an ethical, inductive ("what the facts show") document "lifted" from the crime scene. Any contact with suspects may generate conscious or unconscious prejudice to the extent the profiler modifies the profile to match characteristics observed in the suspect.

2. *Recognizing Evidence.* Training as a forensic investigator with such specific expertise in wound pattern analysis, blood stain patterns, bite mark evidence, and the ability to recognize all physical evidence and how best to interpret, is a must.

3. *Fantasy and Motivation.* All serial crimes have elements of fantasy that fuel the motivation to commit and continue to commit serial crimes. The profiler's job is to reconstruct offender behavior from the physical evidence left behind and look for patterns of psychological value, which illuminate motivation. In trying to apprehend the villain in *Hounds of the Baskervilles,* fictional detective Sherlock Holmes disclosed to Dr. Watson the importance of using imagination to solve crimes. "People will stick to facts even though they lead nowhere . . . but to *imagine what the criminal was thinking and how he might have conceived of the crime* is the key to the criminal mind."

4. *State of Mind.* Was anything brought by the offender to the crime scene such as duct tape, rape kit, blindfold, or handcuffs suggesting premeditation versus spontaneity? Were the stab wounds violent, frenzied, or slashing or were they methodical? Answers to these questions help to uncover the offender's crime scene state of mind.

5. Determine whether or not *modus operandi* and signature "chain" crimes together.

◼ Rival Paradigms

1. United Kingdom Model: Investigative Psychology (IP)

Another systematized attempt to apprehend violent crime offenders is David Cantor's approach to profiling known as *Investigative Psychology* (IP). This model utilizes methods similar to the FBI's statistical use of comparison studies. Statistical analysis of criminal behavior results in the creation of a massive database where offender groups (known as typologies) in Cantor's IP are routinely compared to *known offender populations* to "narrow down" offender characteristics. Known as the Five Factor model, Cantor's perspective focuses on *interactional* aspects between offender and victim.

Know

1. *Interpersonal Coherence*. A tenant of IP purposes that offenders will interact with their victims in similar ways with people in their ordinary, non-criminal interactions. Furthermore, victim selection often represents significant people in the non criminal life of the offender as evidenced by Ted Bundy "selecting" victims that represented his girlfriend.

2. *Significance of Time and Place*. Since the offender *chooses* the time and place of his crimes, this information provides important information regarding the offender's work schedule, possible shift work, time off, and vicinity of residence.

3. *Criminal Characteristics*. Subsystems of criminality used by IP discards "organized" versus "disorganized" characteristics due to the overlap of characteristics of serial offenders. Subsets of criminal behavior—such as educational level, childhood influences, and neighborhood of origin—help to "narrow down" offenders.

4. *Criminal Career*. Assessments made to determine if the offender has a *prior criminal record* suggesting a prior background of burglary, for example, if gaining entrance is easily achieved, or the method of bathing a victim of sexual assault might suggest a prior sexual assault history.

5. *Forensic Awareness*. This component addresses whether or not the offender has *knowledge of forensic evidence* collection such as wearing gloves, "wiping down" evidence, wearing a condom, or removing evidence containing the offender's bodily fluids.

Circle Theory

From Cantor's work in **environmental psychology**, he developed a so-called "circle theory" of offender behavior. Two models have evolved from this theory—the so-called "marauder model" and the "commuter model." Cantor hypothecates that the offender in the "marauder model" will commit offenses close to home (as a trapdoor spider), while in the "commuter model" offenders will travel away from their residence to commit crimes.

2. Behavioral Evidence Analysis

Know

California forensic scientist and private criminal profiler Brent Turvey developed an alternative systemic procedure in profiling violent offenders, in contrast to Cantor's Investigative Psychology and the FBI model.

Turvey's method is known as *Behavioral Evidence Analysis* (BEA). A meticulously prepared investigator, Turvey discovered a curious fact while interviewing incarcerated serial murderer Jerome Brudos. In the face-to-face interview, Brudos *lied about almost all aspects of the crime.* (Turvey would have not known this had he not invested months of "homework" examining investigative reports—court transcripts, forensic reports and other records.)

Behavioral Evidence Analysis seeks to "fill in the gaps" from other systemic approaches. The four steps of Behavioral Evidence Analysis are:

1. *Equivocal Forensic Analysis.* Of all the possible interpretations of crime scene evidence, which one is the *most likely* to be correct? It is imperative to gather all evidence from the crime scene, mull it over, and consider alternative possibilities before deciding on the *best direction* to go. The answer directs the remainder of the profile. Since the initial stage is all about *forensic evidence,* all components of the crime scene must be meticulously investigated by analyzing the following:

    a. crime scene photos
    b. investigative (police) reports
    c. video and photos available from autopsy reports
    d. witness, neighbor interviews
    e. map of victim's travel prior to death
    f. personal background of the victim

Focus on

2. *Victimology.* An in-depth *assessment of the victim* comprises victimology, by consensus one of the most neglected aspects of profiling. According to Turvey, "the why, how, where, when, and why a particular victim was chosen over all others" discloses a great deal of information about the offender. Everything from the victim's body build (**morphology**)—denoting the probable size of the offender—in cases where the body was moved, for example, would shed light on the general strength and size of the offender; ascertaining social skills, adaptability to surroundings, and whether the victim was gullible, and so on, allows investigators to project personality traits in the offender.

3. *Crime Scene Characteristics.* Refers to the distinguishing features of the crime scene relative to the offender's decisions regarding the victim, how the offender likely approached the victim, the choice of location, and how all relevant fact may be tied together in the big picture.

4. *Offender Characteristics.* The preceding steps contribute in producing the single most important domain of information to the profiler: *probable behavioral and personality characteristics of the offender,* which of course, is subject to continual modification as a "running commentary." Step 4 should disclose the offender's

a. morphology
b. sex
c. work status/habits
d. remorse/guilt (or lack of)
e. vehicle type
f. criminal history
g. skill level
h. aggressiveness (or lack of)
i. residence in relation to the crime
j. medical history
k. marital status
l. race/ethnicity

The four stages are further delineated into the *investigative phase,* when violent crimes are initially being committed, and the *trial phase,* where a known suspect sits in the courtroom. The main purpose of the *investigative phase* encompasses:

1. "narrow down" viable suspects,
2. determine if crimes are related,
3. if offender behavior may escalate into more violent crimes,
4. producing leads and strategies to capture, and
5. keeping the investigation robust and on track.

The *trial phase* focuses on:

1. deciding the value and integrity of forensic evidence,
2. developing interviewing or interrogative strategies,
3. gaining insight into offender's state of mind (mens rea) before, during, and after the crime,
4. determining any crime scene evidence suggesting a link to other offenses by virtue of modus operandi and signature

In assessing Turvey's perspective, the quality of the final profile is influenced by the amount of pertinent forensic evidence available, and the inferential skills of the profiler.

In the final analysis, the criminal profile, part art and part science, is an *investigative tool* on par with diagnostic criteria of clinical assessment.

■ In Summation—Alternative Paradigms

Summing up the four approaches discussed in this section, *known offender characteristics* in the vast database of the FBI's computers provide an inductive method of matching crime scene behavior to a highly probable UNSUB. David Cantor's *Investigative Psychology* is driven less by pure forensic evidence and more by principles of psychology, especially *environmental psychology*. Brent Turvey's *Behavioral Evidence Analysis* does not use statistical inferences, but instead relies heavily on *forensic science* to reconstruct the crime and *speculative* (deductive) *logic* in characterizing the players—the behavioral characteristics of both predator and victim.

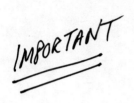

IMPORTANT

■ Species: Pseudo-sapien

As we will show in subsequent chapters by virtue of modern brain scanning technology, neuroscience is already demonstrating in most cases irreversible neurological brain abnormalities in sexual psychopathy manifested not only in adult serial killers, but also in "kids who kill kids and adults—adolescent "Rambo" killers.

Can a neurologically damaged brain leading to *rapacious behavior* be classified without prejudice as truly and authentically homo sapien—a thinking, rational, person who exercises behavioral restraint?

Perhaps damaged cortices in the brains of sexual psychopaths (not garden variety psychopaths) has been "re-wired" so dramatically as a result of the abuse of antisocial parenting and the perverted, aberrant thinking set up by cognitive mapping that sexual psychopathy requires a new sapient classification. Perhaps male and female serial killers and the young "Rambo" killers justify a new moniker precisely because they have a *different brain and neurological system*.

No longer *homo sapien,* characterized by thinking and restraint as *fait accompli* of the species, perhaps **sui generis** designation of **pseudo-sapient** best describes the mind and behavior of human predators who *prey upon others for sexual gratification*.

For sure, a pseudo-sapient brain is not the same brain as normal children, adolescents or adults (even garden variety psychopathy). With the perverted cognitive maps, and unchecked rage careening into sexualized violence, how could it be? In fact, no competent neuropsychologist would suggest the neurologically damaged brain observed in sexual psychopathy to be anywhere near a homo sapien brain. A case in point is the mind of "Boston Strangler" Albert De Salvo.

PREDATOR PROFILE (3-2)

Albert De Salvo
"The Boston Strangler"

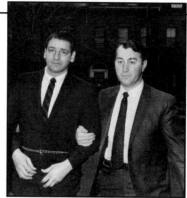
©Bettmann/CORBIS

Alternate Media Monikers:

"The Measuring Man"
"The Green Man"

As a serial killer, Albert De Salvo became known to the world as "The Boston Strangler." De Salvo was born to Frank and Charlotte De Salvo in Boston, Massachusetts. He was raised in Chelsea, MA, which is a poor suburb of working class Boston. In this overcrowded and impoverished area of Boston, Frank was a laborer and a plumber by day, and an abusive husband and father by night. An alcoholic, he physically and mentally abused his children and his wife. Sadly, Frank and his wife had two more sons and three daughters.

Before his father left and the dysfunctional couple divorced, De Salvo watched as his father knocked out his mother's teeth and broke all the fingers on one of her hands. The abuse was extremely harsh on young Albert. At one point in his childhood, De Salvo, along with two of his sisters, were sold as slaves by his father to a farmer for nine dollars. They escaped their "master" in about a month. When he was about six years old, his father introduced him to petty crimes such as shoplifting, which led to burglary, and breaking and entering.

As Albert grew older, his father brought home prostitutes and forced Albert to watch him having sexual intercourse with them. By the age of 10 years old, Albert had already had his first sexual experience. Apparently, having sexual experience at such a young age led to a sexual obsession. Soon, De Salvo became addicted to sex. According to reports, De Salvo claimed to have sex with his wife up to six times a day. According to the DSM, De Salvo could be diagnosed as a sexual sadist, meaning he experienced "recurrent intense sexual urges and sexually arousing fantasies involving acts (real, not simulated) in which the psychological or physical suffering including humiliation (including post mortem) of the victim is sexually exciting to the person."

After high school, De Salvo joined the Army and was sent to Germany. He met and fell in love with a woman he brought back to the states with him. While stationed at Fort Dix, his daughter was born. De Salvo was dishonorably discharged from the Army due to an allegation that he sexually molested a nine-year-old girl. No conviction was obtained due to the mother's failure to file charges against him. After he was discharged, he and his wife moved back to Chelsea where he grew up. De Salvo moved to another suburb of Boston, Malden, MA, where his son was born.

In the late 1950's, De Salvo became a petty criminal by breaking and entering. His wife grew tired of his behavior and soon rejected him. "The Measuring Man" became a media moniker as he stalked young girls, followed them home, and pretended to be a representative of a modeling agency.

He stated he was required to take their physical measurements for the agency to see if they qualified as models. He used his charm to seduce some of the girls into sexual encounters. Even though some girls complained to the police, no authorities intervened. In 1961, De Salvo was arrested for breaking and entering. He spent 11 months in jail. It was after he was released that he turned to murder.

From 1962 until 1964, when De Salvo was arrested, there were 13 victims of his 19-month murder spree. (The term serial killer did not exist at this time.) These murders produced his lasting alias "The Boston Strangler." The vast majority of his early victims were older females, but later he preyed on younger victims before he was eventually caught and sent to jail.

Victimology:

He gained entrance into the homes of his victims by portraying himself as a repairman or someone of authority, such as a police detective. When he started out, he chose only older females. This was believed to be because of a hatred for his mother, or women in general. De Salvo was purported to say

"I did this not as a sex act but out of hate for her. I don't mean out of hate for her in particular, really, I mean out of hate for a woman."

At the end of his criminal career, he started preying on younger victims. He spent little time targeting his victims. All of his victims were sexually molested in some way, and they were strangled with an article of their own clothing. How did De Salvo target his victims?

"Attractiveness had nothing to do with it . . . when this certain time comes on me, it's a very immediate thing. When I get this feeling, instead of going to work I make an excuse to my boss. I start driving and I start building this image up, and that's why I find myself not knowing where I'm going."

Signature:

When he strangled his victims, he tied a bow around their neck with an article of clothing. Not just any bow, but a big floppy bow. He placed the body in an obscene position as to where anyone who entered the apartment after he left would see the victim lying there with no warning. He penetrated the vagina with a foreign object, such as a broom handle or a bottle, or with his penis. It is unclear whether he did this post mortem or while the victim was still alive.

He was arrested on another charge that spawned "The Green Man" alias. Dressed in green trousers, De Salvo was arrested for a string of sexual assaults. These assaults took place over a four state area—Massachusetts, Connecticut, Rhode Island, and New Hampshire. He is believed to have committed over 300 sexual assaults, from which not one of his victims was murdered.

Insanity Plea Fails:

De Salvo's attorney tried to convince the judge and the jury that he had a mental disorder and was not cognizant of the nature of his crimes. He brought in witnesses to testify as to his mental illness. Regardless, he was convicted and sentenced to life at Bridgewater Hospital.

Serial killers are known to be crafty and slippery. Along with two other inmates, De Salvo escaped from the hospital. He was re-captured and moved to a maximum-security prison for the remainder of his sentence. However, six years into his prison term, De Salvo was stabbed through the heart six times in his cell in an apparent prison brawl. His murderer was never identified.

In some comments, De Salvo showed a tinge of remorse for his crimes; however he was also known to brag about them. Therefore, it is hard to tell whether he was being genuine or if he displayed another instance of saying what people wanted to hear. For example in De Salvo's words,

"I would go home and watch what I had done on TV. Then I would cry like a baby."

"If God didn't mean them to be dead they wouldn't be; it was a case of their time being up."

"It (the murders) wasn't as dark and scary as it sounds. I had a lot of fun killing somebody. A funny experience."

① Road Rage Studies
② OutRAGE: O.J. SIMPSON
burnbergs

Aftermath

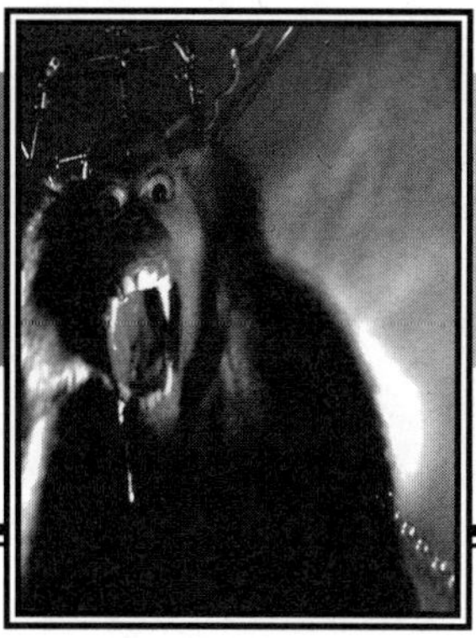

I. Word Scholar

Define the following words from *The Word Scholar Glossary.*

1. Paradigm ______________________________
2. Animism ______________________________
3. Homicidal triad ______________________________
4. Law of association ______________________________
5. Law of effect ______________________________
6. Rapacious ______________________________
7. Cognitive neuroscience ______________________________
8. Dual diagnosis ______________________________
9. Pseudo-sapient ______________________________
10. Necrophilia ______________________________

II. The Forensic Lab

Compose a one page report addressing Jacob's proposed classification of pseudo-sapien referring to brain damaged sexual predators. What is a convincing argument that might compel authorities to view a *sui generis* reclassification of sexual predators?

pseudo sapien — different than homosapien.

new classification

CHAPTER 4

Modus Vivendi—*Sexualized Aspects of Serial Crime: From Fantasy to Aftermath*

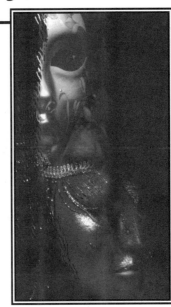

❝*Out of the folds in the back of Mr. Gumb's robe crawled a Death's-head Moth . . . the moth flew. It came from behind him, past his head and lit between them . . . He looked at it. When she didn't look at it, when her eyes never left his face, he knew. Their eyes met and they knew each other . . . She went for the gun . . . 'Freeze.'*❞

—*Silence of the Lambs*
Thomas Harris

Manie sans delire . . .

"By the nineteenth century, *abnormality in the human mind* was being linked to criminal behavior patterns. Philippe Pinel, one of the founders of French psychiatry, claimed that some people *behave abnormally even without being mentally ill.* He coined the phrase *manie sans delire*—"obsession without insanity"—to denote what eventually was referred to as psychopathic personality."

—*Criminology*, L. Siegel

◾ Part I: *Mens Rea*—Criminal Motive, Fantasy, and Eroticism

Chapter Four presents the *five sexualized components of serial crime* from start (with the all-consuming erotic fantasy, forged from an addiction to hardcore pornography, or sexual repression, to finish, with the aftermath, following death. In behavioral psychology, "reading" the mind of a killer is an *inferential* task accomplished by observing behavior, the nature of the crime, the choice of victim, and projecting personality and psychological proclivities into the most likely UNSUB.

Interestingly, Freud was the first maverick personality theorist to use "mind" and "personality" interchangeably. He preferred the term "character disorder" (over personality disorder) in describing long-standing personality deviance. In actuality, Freud's preference better describes the personality of sexual psychopaths. In Freud's view, character is more descriptive of a person's "core of being" than personality; hence, his preference for the word "character" over the word "personality." Believing a person's *character* to be emotionally deviant, then "once a pedophile always a pedophile" and "once a sexual psychopath always a sexual psychopath," reflects ingrained deviance so indelible as to be irreversible. This coincides with modern thinking.

■ How Addiction Works—Through Feeling & Emotion

The author has chosen the Latin term *modus vivendi (MV)* to characterize *sexualized components of rapacious crime*—"*the thrilling high*" connected to *feeling* that is experienced in each murder by the perpetrator. As observed in this chapter and the next, *self-addiction* to his own brain chemistry and hormones is a major factor in feeling "compelled" to continue predatory behavior, rather than cognitively "choosing" the course his action.

Addiction works through emotions and "compels" behavior based on feeling, while a non-addicted and non-mentally ill person makes decisions based on cognition and rationally "choosing" what course to take. In psychopathy, *deviant feelings* trump *cognitive restraint*. In our nomenclature, Homo pseudo-sapiens *feel* their way through one-way relationships with egocentric, rapacious behavior, while Homo sapiens both *think* and *feel* their way through two-way, give-and-take relationships with socially appropriate behavior.

The sexualized aspect of predatory behavior begins with *mens rea*—the criminal motive—with a confusing mix of anger, frustration, fantasy, and perverted erotic desire. In criminal law, *mens rea* is the legal term that comprises the mental "fuse" that ignites the observable behavior of crime.

Motive is derived from the Latin *motus* (pp. of *movere*) meaning, "to move," clearly a verb of action. Motive implies emotion or desire operating on will (cognition) causing action. In this definition, it is *emotion that "wags the tail" of thinking, producing behavior.* Clearly, motivation is "emotional thinking" (sounding like an oxymoron, yet conceptualized as "heart over head").

Selection of the victim (organized offender), or crossing the path of an unfortunate victim (disorganized offender), reflects a human predator deep into sexualized fantasies, anger, frustration, and perverted eroticism—a perplexing cocktail of circulating neurochemistry that *compels,* that drives, sequential rape and murder. To the serial killer, murderous thoughts gravitate around *emotion*—the feeling that comes with complete domination, degradation, and sexual experimentation of the victim. Sadly, it's the only thing that "jazzes" him in his otherwise depressing life.

Following discussion of the sexualized motivation inherent in criminal intent (*mens rea*), the remaining elements will be discussed, which are: the physical act of murder *actus reus* (and corresponding components of *actus reus,* namely *modus operandi* and signature), and aftermath, following the death of the victim.

The study of motivation has always intrigued psychology. From the classic studies of Abraham Maslow's *hierarchy of needs* and McClelland's *achievement motivation* to the celebrated **Hawthorne Effect** of Elton Mayo in his "Western Electric Studies," researchers gained insight into human motivation. Blue chip companies pay **I/O psychologists** six and seven figure dollar amounts to motivate employees toward higher profits against fierce competition. In forensic psychology and criminology, knowledge of motive (and *signature*) often separates the exceptional profiler from the average one.

Always an element, *sexualized motivation* may not be obvious at the crime scene, but it's the first thing on the mind of an experienced profiler.

◼ Sexualized *Mens Rea*

Sexual fantasies, and the behavior leading to the kill (similar to sexual foreplay) jazzes the serial predator's perverted emotional life like no other, yet, ultimately, only temporarily. As Bundy noted the "brutal urge" always comes back stronger.

Sexualized fantasies, spawned from an addiction to **pornography, voyeurism,** and/or *fetishism,* enhanced by alcohol or drug addiction (what we have termed poly-addiction) provide the emotional "fuse" of *mens rea.* Upon capture, serial killers are often arrogant and unremorseful. They are not sorry for committing crimes; rather, they are sorry they got caught. Psychologically tethered to chaos or havoc in their personal lives, it is a sad irony that serial murderers try in vain to gain a measure of control by dominating, humiliating, and ultimately killing others.

The more serial killers "succeed" in victimizing others, the more addicted they become to their scary, inner world of sexual exploitation fueled by an addiction to hardcore, violent pornography, or in the alternative, an all-consuming sexual repression leading (as in the case of Ed Gein) to pathological curiosity. According to the FBI's study of serial homicide, the *most common thread running through all serial killers is an addiction to hardcore pornography.* As sexual tension builds from his full-blown "porn" compulsion, the serial predator is ever eager to apply what he has learned from his last murder by plotting the next one. Compulsively watching pornography keeps sexual tension high. The organized serial killer becomes **obsessive-compulsive** in his macabre fascination with sexual exploitation through rape and murder.

Through journal entries, and/or "trophies"—articles of the victim's clothing, a bracelet, or a shoe, or sometimes in bizarre instances of cannibalism, a body part (Jeffrey Dahmer favored the victim's head)—the killer keeps souvenirs of the crime. By "crossing the line" and committing the first homicide, most serial killers remained compelled to kill again and again, much like the addict becomes addicted to his drug of choice.

Although somewhat rare, a few offenders become overwhelmed with the emotional realization of the severity of the crime and find themselves apprehensive as if "begging" to get caught. However, this is extremely rare.

◼ Isolation Drives *Mens Rea*

As mentioned in Chapter Two, the developmental psychologist Erik Erikson targets the crisis of *intimacy* versus *isolation* as a major influence in young adults (20 to mid-30 years of age), the age most populated by serial predators. Merging Erikson's theory with brain neuroscience, perhaps the neurologically deficient brain is on a collision with outrage due to *feeling lonely, isolated, and emotionally disconnected.*

Perhaps Erikson would agree that the serial offender's sexual fantasies are too **dissonant** for his damaged brain and lack of experience to bridle predatory thinking. He may feel overwhelmed with a final insult of feeling *isolation* from those around him—"no one understands." Perhaps his only comfort comes from the quick "fix" of compulsive masturbation and fantasy; there's always the fantasy.

To further elucidate the critical importance of developmental stages in psychopathy, Erikson's stages of psychosocial development are presented in more detail in Chapter Five.

In Predator Profile (4-1) we meet Richard Ramirez, "The Night Stalker." His one adult mentor was his "pot"smoking uncle, a Vietnam veteran, who delighted in recalling his sexual conquests and brutality towards others during his tour of duty. Ramirez began his life of crime as a voyeur, rapist, and finally, a serial killer.

[handwritten margin note:] Lack of connection. No understanding of family. Feeling of Isolation.

PREDATOR PROFILE (4-1)

Richard Ramirez
"The Night Stalker"

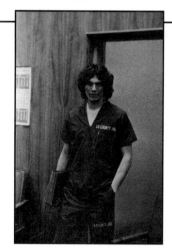

©Bettmann/CORBIS

Like most serial killers, Richard Ramirez's childhood was far from functional. Absent parental competence, he never received the care and love expected in rearing healthy children. A serious epileptic condition was never properly addressed as he suffered numerous seizures.

The one adult mentor in his life, his uncle, was marijuana addicted and a Vietnam veteran. He bragged to young Richard about his brutalities and sexual conquest during the war. Ramirez received a steady "diet" of Polaroid snapshots of rape and killing from his uncle's macabre achieves of war. Richard's uncle taught young Richard how to fight to kill. One afternoon while Richard was visiting his uncle, his uncle shot his wife in the face with a pistol as they fought over his "pot" smoking habit.

In high school, the path became broader for Ramirez to become a serial killer. In his job cleaning hotel rooms, he often broke into rooms to watch guests undress. His first offense of rape occurred when he surprised a hotel guest in her room, tied her up, and began to assault her. Fortuitously, the victim's husband interrupted the crime, catching Ramirez in the act and turning him over to the police. Since Ramirez was only 15 years of age, the judge reduced his punishment to probation (a judicial *faux pas* that enabled Ramirez to continue his crime spree).

Later, Ramirez began using the mind-altering drug, **LSD (lysergic acid diethylamide)** that, no doubt, enhanced his belief that he was merging into one with Satan. His favorite song, Night Prowler, from the rock group AC/DC, further fueled his deviant fantasies.

In 1984, he broke into the home of a seventy-nine year-old widow. He raped and killed her. Subsequently, he murdered fifteen more individuals. Miraculously, many of his victims survived to describe their ordeal. His MO reflected the behavior of a *disorganized* serial rapist/murder. On August 31, 1985, while trying to steal a car from a screaming woman, a mob of onlookers interceded and prevented the hijacking. During his arrest, Ramirez gave a rambling, chilling testimony of his behavior . . .

> ". . . I love to kill people. I love watching them die. I would shoot them in the head and they would wiggle and squirm all over the place, and then just stop. Or I would cut them with a knife and watch their face turn real white. I love all that blood . . . I told one lady to give me all her money. She said 'no,' so I cut her and pulled her eyes out."

He was later convicted of 13 murders. He was sentenced to death and now resides as a death row inmate.

Modus Operandi:

Ramirez's method was to break and enter a home and surprise his sleeping victims. If he found a boyfriend or husband, he used a small .25 caliber pistol to shoot him in the head. He then proceeded to rape his female victim. Often, he would cut her throat to further sexualize the crime. On other occasions, he would beat the victim unconscious and leave her to die.

Signature:

The way Ramirez used violence by ravaging his victims—beating them, slitting their throat, and disfiguring them after death—comprised his signature. He once carved the AC/DC symbol on one of his victims.

Student Contributors:

Jeff Barker and Michelle Heins, PA

◼ Part II of Modus Vivendi: *Actus Reus*— The Criminal Act

Ignited by sexualized fantasy (*mens rea*) gained from his secret porno-graphic archives, it is the physical act, the *actus reus*—the act of murder—that brings law enforcement into the orbit of serial killers. From a young age, we are taught we are free to think any thoughts we want without consequences, but acting on them is another story.

In criminal law, the term *actus reus* denotes the physical component—the criminal act—that constitutes *serious crimes against persons* (**malum in se** crimes from British common law). In sexualized crimes, *actus reus* is characterized by violating the victim's body by the perpetrator's penis, fingers, hands, knives, ligatures, or other objects that inflict torture, pain, and/or death.

In murder by firearm, *actus reus* is the simple act of *pulling* the trigger; in a stabbing death, it's slashing, plunging, or thrusting *motions* of the knife. In ligature (garrote) strangulation, it's the *motions* required in tying the knot or *pressure* on the tourniquet resulting in death. In sexualized crime, perpetrators *seek to prolong actus reus* as long as possible. Ironically, the sexual behavior of serial killers during *actus reus* can be eerily compared to the *foreplay phase* of the human sexual response. Sustaining this stage as along as possible prolongs the killer's erotic fantasies. It's a vital part of the *addiction factor* of serial rape and murder.

◼ Fantasy & Erotic Cognitive Maps

According to sexual researchers (Hendrick & Hendrick, 1992), unless consenting partners *feel safe* in sexual encounters, they will not be fully and comfortably receptive of intercourse or sexual pleasuring. To the serial killer intent upon sexual exploitation, his need for control, domination, degradation, and manipulation replaces receptivity to intimacy in consensual sex.

Because *serial killers are sexual perverts,* they are motivated to find victims to sexually exploit. Sexually perverted *cognitive maps*—powerful "thinking maps" that lie behind sexual fantasies—inexorably lead to murder (*actus reus*). By contrast, normal, healthy, neurological development produces balanced neurochemistry and hormones. These conditions produce far different "maps" of erotic thoughts than the neurologically damaged brain of the sexual psychopath whose violent, hardcore *pornographic eroticism* is the single most damaging component.

In strikingly similar ways, the *four-stage model of sexual arousal* by classic sex researchers Masters and Johnson offer insight into the sexualized crimes of the serial killer.

◼ The Human Sexual Response and Sexualized Crime—Striking Similarities

According to Masters and Johnson, the first stage of the human sexual response is the **excitement phase** prompted by erotic thoughts, sights, or physical contact. The most marked aspect of the excitement phase in males is vasocongestion of blood in three spongy cylinders—two *corpora cavernosa* on the top of the penis and one *corpus spongiosum* on the bottom—resulting in penile erection.

It is not unusual to assume an extended, multi-layered period of the excitement phase occurring in serial rapists and killers. First, erotic fantasy fueled by pornography is partially responsible for targeting a victim. Then, the search begins. Sexually jazzed, they drive around in neighborhoods, perhaps unfamiliar to them, all the while searching, fantasizing, and anticipating. As a victim is targeted, the excitement phase may peak and become almost unbearable to the serial predator, who has spent vast amounts of time in preparation. If he fears being seen so that capture is forestalled, he may masturbate in his car. If possible, he may get close to her in a crowd of people and brush up against her in a brief moment of **frottage**.

The **plateau stage** of Masters and Johnson is equivalent to feeling that the sexual act is imminent. Physiologically, males experience intense muscular tension and full erection. To the serial rapist or killer, as fantasy transitions into confronting the victim, the plateau stage compels the serial predator to move forward and capture her with *actus reus*. In the plateau phase, rapists and killers often *take as much time as possible preparing the victim* for rape or murder, once they have incapacitated victims with handcuffs, ligature or **rape kit**. Just like lovers in a sexual frenzy, the killer begins his sexual siege.

In Masters and Johnson, the **orgasmic phase** is the summit of the human sexual response cycle, characterized by orgasm, ejaculation, and release of muscular tension, even though it lasts no more than 15–20 seconds. The serial killer's orgasmic phase—the expenditure and release of sexual tension—may occur during any or all of the following:

1. rape,
2. fondling,
3. masturbation,
4. stabbing,
5. ligature strangulation,
6. beating,
7. vaginal/anal intercourse,
8. sodomy,
9. sadism,
10. fetishism, or
11. overkill (mutilation).

Many serial killers have admitted to criminal investigators the dread they experience in killing victims, because death brings to an end the *highly anticipated* plateau and orgasmic phases (unless necrophilia is highly prized). For example, Jeffrey Dahmer experimented with "living zombies" as sex slaves by pouring acid into holes he drilled into victims' skulls hoping to keep them alive for continued sexual experimentation.

The final stage, or aftermath, following orgasm is the **resolution phase** in Masters and Johnson's human sexual response. Physiologically, the body returns to its pre-arousal state. Muscle tension subsides, and all physiological responses return to normal, such as heart rate, breathing, and blood pressure. In Ted Bundy's words the "brutal urge" to touch, to control, to penetrate the victim in *sexualized signature,* finally subsides.

Given an array of choices, Halpern & Sherman (1979) suggest that normal sexual partners prefer to touch in the resolution phase. In contrast, the serial killer experiences increasing sexual tension as he kills his victim; he may continue to brutalize the corpse (overkill) following rape or murder. In instances of **necrophilia**, he continues to have sex with the corpse long after his victim is dead. He may return days later and continue.

■ Part III of Modus Vivendi: *Modus Operandi (MO)*

Step-By-Step Procedures within *Actus Reus*

According to Jacobs (2003), *Modus operandi* (MO in police and FBI lingo) is the third component of modus vivendi—the sexualized components of serial crime. Part of actus reus, MO, reflects typical physical methods and procedures the killer uses as he proceeds, step-by-step, with the crime. (In contrast to MO, signature *personalizes* the state of *emotional attachment* to the crime for a specific perpetrator).

MO is a legalistic term denoting the perpetrator's *physical procedures—step by step—*during the commission of the crime. MO is "how" he did it.

In rapacious crimes, MO is a function of learning, experience, and modifications employed from feedback at the crime scene. Hence, it is not surprising to find MO to be *routinely modified* as perpetrators gain more experience and confidence. Organized serial predators are very astute observers; they pay particular attention to every detail of the crime; they are meticulous to a fault with crime scene feedback. According to Ressler and Douglas, this is not the case with the *disorganized* offender whose MO, if any, is haphazard.

■ Dynamics of MO

MO exists as a dynamic, hence changeable, quality that develops over time. For example, in his first crime, a serial offender learns from direct experience how difficult it is to prevent his victim from screaming; he uses what's available at the crime scene such as a sock or piece of cloth forced into her mouth.

Subsequent crimes may show the offender "graduated" to a "**rape kit**"—consisting of duct tape, rope, or other supplies he needs to render the victim helpless. At best, MO shows the evolution of a given predator's step-by-step *actus reus;* hence it is important to note that by itself, due to its evolving nature, *MO is not an accurate gauge in apprehending serial predators.*

■ Shaping Criminal Behavior

Behavioral psychology uses the following terms to explain how experience provides feedback to "shape and maintain" learned behavior:

1. **successive approximations,**
2. **shaping,** and
3. **chaining**

Small steps and chaining evolve into shaped behavior—the final product of behavior—as evidence by MO within *actus reus.*

Applying behavioral psychology to serial crimes, the *small steps* taken by the offender during the commission of his crime comprise the *successive approximations* of the final, end result of death. For example, the period of time used by a predator for *voyeurism*—watching a targeted victim, followed by careful documentation of "comings and goings"—gives him the best time and best place to commit the crime. As serial killer Ted Bundy admitted in an interview, "the victim may not know the perpetrator, but the perpetrator certainly knows the victim."

Careful analysis by the offender may disclose the best way to enter a targeted residence is through a window in the back of the property located away from heavily traveled streets. Wearing a ski mask helps to prevent detection, or deciding on the best way to surprise the sleeping victim are methods used to accomplish the crime comprising his *successive approximations*—the summation of all the small steps used. When the *small steps* of MO are put together into a sequence, a seamless "chaining" of behavior produces *shaping—the behavioral sequence* that produced the crime scene.

Unless the entire process is observed, every specific step taken by the killer in the commission of the total crime (including aftermath), investigators never know with certainty the entire process. However, due to the accuracy of statistical analysis and crime re-construction using computer models, investigators usually gather enough information to construct an accurate profile. Upon being apprehended, the offender often addresses the evolution of procedures that characterized his MO.

■ Experience: The Best Teacher

MOs may be relatively unchanged in one aspect of the crime but "evolved" in other aspects. For example, entering a window, late at night, wearing a ski mask to prevent identification, and away from a busy parking lot, may remain the baseline MO for a serial rapist entering the bedroom of a victim and gagging her with a piece of clothing. However, committing crimes in single family dwelling versus an apartment complex is an instance of an MO not likely to change. An offender who is comfortable attacking victims in a home with less exposure to other people, versus an apartment with "paper-thin walls", will likely continue in his "comfort zone."

Authorities realize the extent most offenders go through in the development of MO and the immense amount of time devoted to each crime from fantasy to aftermath. Imagine how serial predators' lives could have been different had they used all the energy expended in rapacious behavior into building productive careers or healthy relationships. The glaring problem here, of course, is they don't know the first thing about normalcy.

◾ Part IV of *Modus Vivendi*: Signature

"Calling Card" within *Actus Reus*

In contrast to MO, **signature** (or **personation**) is the predator's emotional *cri de coeur*—"cry from the heart", denoting the killer's emotional connection to his victim and the nature of his predatory behavior at the crime scene. Signature is *ritualistic behavior* at the crime scene, suggesting the *underlying emotional theme,* or motive. Not necessary to the commission of the crime, signature is the offender's personal, sexualized, "imprint" exemplified in verbalization or behavior that is *typical and distinguishable* versus all other offenders.

For example, a serial rapist's graphic vocalization may be his signature. Typical and distinguishable at every crime scene, he may intimidate and humiliate his victims with very graphic, degrading, and vulgar talk. He may force victims to say something vulgar in each incidence of rape, such as "I know you've fantasized about this before." Signature is disclosed when he forces his victim to perform the same sexual act in a certain sequence, such as performing oral sex on him and at orgasm, he ejaculates on her stomach or breasts. This instance of signature allows crimes to be linked together as forensic evidence against a targeted offender. As we have seen, behavioral psychologists refer to behavior that is "linked" together in a certain sequence, as *chaining,* or chained behavior).

An entirely different signature occurs, for instance, when a serial rapist enters as a burglary suspect and as soon as he disables his victim and gains control by handcuffing her, he morphs into the "rapist mode." He may force her to masturbate herself at gunpoint while he masturbates himself, and then ejaculates into her vaginally. The first example versus the latter instance shows how two different serial rapists display two different signatures.

◾ Sexualized Signature: The Fantasy Element

At the crime scene, the presence of *signature is perhaps the best justification for characterizing serial crimes as sexualized.* Never changing (but perhaps escalating) signature remains a constant and enduring part of the offender's *behavioral dynamics* and is linked more to the psychological elements—the "fantasy elements"—often expressed in graphic sexual behavior or in sexual overtones. In addition, signature may not always show up at all crime scenes due to unexpected interruptions or unanticipated victim behavior.

In serial homicides, a killer's signature may be bloody attacks seen as **overkill**, where he slashes his victims' bodies with multiple stab wounds or other mutilations, or instances of "graffiti"—initials, words, or symbols cut into victims' bodies—which are all unnecessary in causing death, hence the term *overkill*. Whatever aspect of *actus reus* not necessary to killing the victim may be viewed as signature. For example, after death some victims are placed in certain positions with certain body parts exposed (usually one her breasts) in curious **tableaux mortido** (death pictures)—situated in meticulous detail, evidence of the need to dominate and control, specific traits found in serial offenders.

Analysis of crime scene evidence shows that offenders spend considerable time at the crime scene as though prolonging their murderous fantasies as long as possible, just as normal lovers seek to prolong sexual encounters by touching, cuddling, or sleeping together.

Forensically, signature provides the "stake in the heart" in the conviction of the serial killers, as crimes are linked together by the "smoking gun" of signature analysis. Experienced field agents in local law enforcement and the FBI can attest that the odds of two different offenders fitting the same MO and signature, while operating in the same area at the same time, is remote.

Experienced profilers, such as Ressler and Douglas, suggest that when the "how" of actus reus (the MO) and the "why" of actus reus (the signature) are connected, the "who" (the serial killer) is targeted.

To the forensic psychologist, it is instructive to analyze, understand, and document, in as much detail as possible, *crime scene dynamics*—the elements of *modus vivendi* covered thus far—*mens rea, actus reus, modus operandi, and signature*. The aftermath of the crime—the time subsequent to death—is the fifth factor of *modus vivendi*.

In behavioral psychology, the **law of frequency** states the more frequently a person (e.g. serial killer) makes a response to a given stimulus (stalking and killing a victim), the more likely he will make the same response to the same stimuli in the future (continue serial killing). In other words, this behavioral law accounts for one of the most recognizable idioms in pop culture—"practice makes perfect."

The *law of frequency* explains why serial killers practice what they fantasize; they seek perfection in the macabre practice of death. Another prescient behavioral law, the **law of recency**, states that the more recent a response was made to a given stimulus, the more likely it will be made again—very soon.

■ Part V of *Modus Vivendi*—Aftermath

The period following any ruinous event is known as **aftermath**. In the aftermath of serial rape or murder, the perpetrator may perform **necrophilia**—sexual intercourse with the corpse—or other sexualized behavior demonstrating the macabre "relationship" envisioned by the killer to his victim. For example, serial killer Jeffrey Dahmer anticipated lying next to his victims and later cannibalizing some part of the victim's body as a way to feel "connected"; a way to make him a part of his body forever.

Numerous killers returned to perform sexual acts with the corpses or parts of the corpses. Reliving the rape and/or murder extends the "thrilling high" and allows the perpetrator to savor the sexualized feeling. He may revisit the crime scene, a shallow burial spot or cemetery, so the sexualized elements associated with fantasy and the crime itself can be experienced one more time.

▪ Contrasting *Modus Operandi* & Signature: A Student Profiler's Perspective

MO is defined as any action or series of actions performed by a perpetrator as a necessary means of accessing and/or isolating the victim. Here, the mental, fantasy part (*mens rea*) becomes actualized. Any aspects of MO can be refined, improved, or even discarded as required by serial killers to achieve their goal of acquiring victims, disabling them and raping and/or killing them. The following are examples of *modus operandi*:

1. Use of **ruses** (romancing, flirtation, asking for help)

2. Stalking, or otherwise locating a *particular type* of victim
       Targeting a prostitute, hitchhiker, student, or ground floor resident
       Specificity of body build, hair color, gender, age, race

3. Choosing a certain location:
       May be significant to the perpetrator
       Easy access to the victim
       Permits escape from the crime scene
       Satisfies requirements of signature

4. Use of restraints, force, or a weapon to incapacitate, restrain, silence, and/or kill the victim.

Signature

Signature is defined as any action or series of actions performed by a perpetrator that is *not necessary* to raping or killing her during and/or after the physical commission of a crime. *Emotionality* enters *actus reus* and becomes *personalized with signature*. Signature is unique to each killer, such as:

1. Verbalizations made to the victim.
2. Apologizing to the victim.
3. Ante-mortem or post-mortem sexual activity with or without the victim (rape, masturbation, necrophilia).
4. Taking of trophies (body parts, locks of hair, jewelry).

5. Ante-mortem or post-mortem markings, mutilation, or dismemberment (overkill).
6. Washing of the corpse.
7. "Staging" of the corpse.
8. Returning to the crime scene or grave of the victim.
9. Joining the investigatory process.

Criminal Math

Mens Rea + Actus Reus + (MO & Signature) = Corpus Delicti

In serial crimes, mens rea (criminal, mental intent) plus actus reus (MO and signature) equals corpus delicti, or the body of forensic evidence required by prosecuting attorneys to move forward in court. Additionally, signature is essential for analysis in order to connect crimes together perpetrated by the same offender.

Student Contributor: Rea Ellen Wooten, PA

In conclusion, similar to consensual sex between lovers, serial killers *sexualize every phase of the crime* against his victim from (1) fantasy—including the search, confrontation, and capture of the victim to (2) the physical acts during the attack (*actus reus*), including (2a) *modus operandi* (MO)—how he proceeds with his method of physically making the crime happen, to (2b) signature (his emotional *cri de coeur,* and finally to (3) aftermath, which may or may not involve overkill, necrophilia, or **staging**—placing the body in a particular position in anticipation of being discovered by authorities.

■ The Phenomenon of Staging

Staging refers to actions by the perpetrator or other persons that *purposely alters the crime scene* prior to the arrival of the police. Investigators know staging takes place for at least two reasons:

1. The perpetrator purposively manipulates the crime scene attempting to direct the *investigation away from the most logical suspect—himself.* Being overly cooperative or ostentatiously distraught, perpetrators attempt to steer the investigation to other more "logical" suspects.

2. A family member tries to protect the victim (and/or the victim's family). This occurs predominantly in *rape-murder crimes* or **autoerotic** fatalities (such as **autoerotic asphyxiation**) when a family member or friend discovers the body first. Perpetrators in rape-murder crimes often leave the body in curious *tableaux* that is shocking and/or degrading. Hence, staging in this instance would be an attempt to leave some

dignity to the victim as observed when a husband covers his wife's nude body, or a wife cuts down her husband from the noose following accidental death due to an autoerotic episode. The wife may try to make her husband's death in such a case look like a suicide. She may even go as far as to write a suicide note. (Middle aged and older males may have a stroke or heart attack and die while masturbating to pornographic movies. Wives will remove the pornographic videos from the residence as well as any evidence of his autoerotic behavior in an instance of staging a non-criminal related event.)

"Red Flags" of Staging

Inconsistencies between crime scene analysis and evidence, and the position of the body in reference to context in the overall picture, leads to "red flags" of staging and aids in the prevention of a "misdiagnosis" of the crime scene. Point of entry, point of exit, time of day, and other evidence exist as "red flags" alerting investigators to potential discrepancies.

Suppose a homeowner returns home from work and interrupts an attempted burglary. The startled burglar kills the man in his own home. An inventory of the crime scene discloses the burglar did not steal anything of value, such as easily accessible jewelry or expensive electronic equipment. Using *skepticism* and *speculative logic,* analyze *alternative theories* suggested by the following as to why the man was killed.

1. Unfortunately, the man startled the burglar, leading to his death; the burglar simply fled the residence without stealing anything.
2. The "burglar" was not a burglar at all.
3. The wife was involved.
4. The wife and "burglar" staged the whole "burglary attempt." They were secretly having an affair. She and the burglar staged the crime to kill the husband and make it appear to be a bungled burglary.

◼ Skepticism

Psychologically, the experienced profiler approaches a crime scene by philosophical **skepticism**—the "mindset" of withholding opinions until all the facts have been gathered and analyzed. An example of the failure to use skepticism (educated doubt) occurred in the recent events surrounding the sniper attacks in Virginia (2002). Nightly news "talking heads" attempted to profile the individual with very limited information. When the snipers were eventually captured, the profiles proved to be misleading and wrong. On a nationally syndicated program, experienced FBI profiler Greg McCrary later spoke out against hasty attempts to profile offenders on limited information. In the snipers' case, McCrary noted there simply was not enough evidence to produce an accurate profile.

◨ Psychology of Sexual Sadism— Psychopathology of Compliant Victims

From the pioneering work of former FBI agent Roy Hazelwood, accurate insight into the mind of sexual sadists and their compliant victims—a female co-offender who helps "recruit" other victims for her sadist "lover"—is being systematized. **Sexual sadism** is defined as a sexual perversion where gratification is obtained by the infliction of a physical, sexual nature with accompanying mental anguish.

In many cases of sexual sadism, *victims are kept alive as long as possible* to prolong the perverse sexual appetites of the sadist. The *fait accompli* of serial sexual sadism is rape or murder. (The word "sadist" is derived from the exploits of the nineteenth century *Marquis de Sade,* a count that delighted in inflicting sexual cruelties on his "lovers.") According to Hazelwood, five steps by the sadist are observed in the "creation" of his perverse "female Igor"—the **compliant co-offender**. The steps are:

1. Through astute observation of **body language**, the sadist identifies a *vulnerable* co-offender—a female who is naïve, dependent, immature and therefore, controllable. Often, such a compliant person has a diagnosable **dependent personality disorder** already displaying behavior consistent with co-dependency—being a "doormat" for others. She may have come from parents who were abusive, or from an abusive relationship with a boyfriend or ex-husband. In any event, the sadist appears as the "saving" persona, her "rescuer".

2. The sadist charms her with his "smooth talk" and seemingly gentle nature. He may lavish her with gifts, offer physical protection, financial support, or whatever he perceives necessary as the "legitimate" answer to her problems. The victim perceives him as a loving and caring "nurturer," worthy of her love. Women often "fall" for the demeanor and **persona** (social "masks" used by psychopathic individuals for the purpose of deception).

3. Soon, totally dependent upon him and under his emotional "spell," she in encouraged to *engage in perverse sexual practices* she most likely considers to be deviant or at the very least "kinky." The *small steps* he uses to lure her into his perverse world eventually leads to *shaping* full-blown perversities, soon evolving into habitual sexual practices. The shaping of sexual perversity accomplishes two control mandates, one—demolishes her fragile will and "esteem" and any sense of normalcy regarding values, and two—the *fait accompli* of sexual sadism, *isolation from others.* After a relatively short time, the co-offender becomes a sexual "slave." With a compliant co-offender, the sadist perversely gets "his cake and eats it, too".

4. Through domination, manipulation, control, and physical punishment for lapses, the sadist becomes the center of the "recruit's" universe. The compliant co-offender feels hopeless and depersonalized, which will eventually play a central role in victimization. Sadly, she is worse off in the hands of the sadist than in any prior dysfunctional relationship.

Through *mind control* and *physical punishment,* she complies with his every demand, partly to avoid his wrath. He has succeeded in her new cognitive map "make-over." As mentioned early, powerful cognitive maps provide the blueprint for self-concept, feeling, and behavior. The sadist has reduced her fragile (or non-existent self-esteem) into the persona of a "bad," "stupid," "inferior," or "inadequate", "depersonalized" slave. She is a pure example of **co-dependency.**

◼ Signature Sexual Offenders—Sadist Signature Killers

Criminologist, homicide detective, and true crime author Robert Keppel (*Signature Killers* 1997) presents his own paradigm to explain the slowly developing sadistic homicide offenders—his term is *signature killers*—due to the unmistakable presence in all crime scenes of his sadistic "calling card."

Mentioned earlier, signature relates to motive, emotionality, and ultimately, sexualized "non-fulfillment," according to Ressler and others. The *addictionologist* knows why serial predators are *compelled* to *continue criminal behavior;* they operate out of a full-blown addiction where every aspect of the crime is sexualized.

According to Keppel, the basis for understanding even the most minor of sex offenses (in his words "Sex Crimes 101") is the realization that serial killers are *driven by anger expressed through control.* Keppel uses the following categories in analyzing serial crimes by describing *psychological dynamics* within the perpetrator manifested at the crime scene:

1. *The Anger-Retaliation Signature.* Driven by anger toward his victim who he symbolically uses as *retaliation against the source of his anger,* this signature often displays *overkill* as the victim becomes an anger-retaliation symbol. Examples of serial killers who follow this typology include Arthur Shawcross and John Wayne Gacy. According to Shawcross, he murdered women because his mother rejected him, while Gacy murdered "lost boys" who sought consolation from him. He retaliated against them as a symbol for his hatred of his alcoholic father who never expressed genuine emotion and love. (The reason serial killers are so dangerous is that they are not what they appear to be. Serial killers may pose as roofers or service technicians as they canvass victims door to door. They may return several months later in what appears to be a random, chance occurrence, or they may dress as a clown—as Gacy did—to entertain children.) The anger-retaliation killer seldom kills his own mother; he chooses someone like her. Victims are chosen who represent domineering women in their lives whom they portray as responsible for their troubles, unless the killer is homosexual and seeks to destroy young males. According to Keppel, examples include mothers who were over-controlling, promiscuous, physically or sexually abusive, or mothers who inspired fear and terror in her children, or fathers who rejected their sons.

[handwritten note:] Jerry Blair — could reflect their dissatisfaction they feel within themselves manifested outwardly through rage towards their victim.

2. *The Picquerism Signature.* The serial killer who is a picquerist is a sexual deviant who is sexually aroused by penetration of the skin by cutting, slicing, or stabbing with a long-bladed knife, or biting the victim. In rare cases, picquerism may involve sniper activity. Victims are not victims of chance. Victims are chosen because they fit the killer's preferred type. He may stalk his victim for weeks or months. (The results of picquerist crimes are particularly gruesome due to deep and violent stab wounds. *Penetration by a knife blade and controlling every aspect of bringing death to his victims* drives this type of signature homicide.) After six picquerist murders near San Diego, California, a twenty-five year old black male, Cleophus Price, was identified as the serial killer.

3. *Sexual Sadism Signature.* According to Dr. Richard Walter, a forensic psychologist at Michigan State Penitentiary, the three Ds of sexual sadism are *dread, dependency, and degradation.* Prolonging the sexual "high" in each stage by inflicting as much pain and misery as possible provides the killer with *modus vivendi*—sexualized feelings related to sadism such as breaking his victim's *will to resist* him. Delaying the death of the victim prolongs the sadist's desire for psychological terrorism. If death comes too fast, the serial sexual sadist feels cheated.

◼ The Sexual Addiction Factor

More importantly, *signature* provides evidence of the *addiction factor* that highlights serial rapes and murders, according to Jacobs (2003). Due to many factors relative to learning and neurochemistry, offenders are addicted to the feeling—the "thrilling high" generated in the brain's *pleasure pathways.* The same pathways explain addiction to any drug, such as alcohol, marijuana, cocaine, or MDMA (ecstasy). Although some serial killers dreaded killing the victim, *restraining the victim* and controlling when the victim dies produced more of the "thrilling high" than murder.

The relentless *addiction factor* compelling serial killers from one kill to another is what Bundy called the "brutal urge", only to feel it recede by feeling "spent" in aftermath. The words used to describe his addiction could have been used to describe two lovers tearing off each other's clothes and having consensual sex in a wild display of shared passion. To the *organized* serial offender, the parallels are striking. This comes as startling news to so-called "experts" who interject decision into the motivation of serial psychopaths. They are ignorant of the psychological ramifications of addiction and neurochemistry that lie behind emotion. Serial crime is driven by feeling, not cognitive decision-making.

To forensic neuroscientists studying serial rape and homicide, the most important ingredients to be addressed are:

1. The driving force of erotic *feeling* relative to his sexual fantasies as he *contemplates* the crime,
2. How he *feels* (as *mens rea* accelerates) *preparing* to commit the crime,
3. How *feeling* carries him through the physical perpetration of full-blown *actus reus* exemplified in MO and signature, and
4. How he *feels* "spent" with endorphin release in aftermath.

To the neuroscientist, every step from imagery to debauchery to aftermath is due to neurochemistry and neurohormones driven by fantasies, deviant cognitive "mapping," reaching climax in MO and signature. This view explains why some serial killers are repulsed by the memory of the crime the next morning when alcohol (or other drugs) wears off. But, as Bundy explained in his last interview prior to lethal injection, the "brutal urge" always comes back.

Proposed neurochemical underpinnings behind rapacious behavior detailed in Chapter Five provides compelling evidence that serial killers' cognitive "decision" to rape or murder is due more to *feeling compelled* by his *chemical addiction* (to his own brain chemistry and/or poly-addiction to other drugs) acting as a compulsion as a means to act out what he has already fantasized. Compelled by addiction makes more sense to the neuroscientist than a rational, cognitive decision to kill—the so-called "choice" serial offenders are presumed to make because of rage, anger, or retribution for past ignoble influences.

◾ Paraphilias

The essential features of **paraphilias** are recurrent, intense sexually arousing fantasies, sexual urges, or behaviors generally involving the following:

1. Non-human objects
2. Sadism: Causing the emotional suffering of another
3. **Masochism:** Causing emotional humiliation
4. **Pedophilia:** Sexualizing children (or other non-consenting persons)

◾ Voyeurism

In the early developmental stages of a serial killer, he may show signs of a sexual deviance known as voyeurism. *Voyeurism* is characterized by the act of observing unsuspecting individuals, usually strangers, who are naked, in the process of becoming naked, or engaging in sexual behavior. The act of looking or "peeping" (Peeping Tom) is for the purpose of *achieving sexual excitement,* and generally no sexual activity with the observed person is sought. Convicted killer Richard Ramirez began his serial killer "career" by observing hotel guests in various stages of nudity.

In its severest form, peeping constitutes the exclusive form of observing sexual activity as *Peeping Toms.* Voyeurism causes clinically significant distress or social or occupational impairment in the voyeur, unless the voyeur is a sexual psychopath. Voyeurism is designated 302.82 in the DSM.

◾ Frotteurism

Frotteurism is characterized by touching or rubbing against a non-consenting person. The behavior usually occurs in crowded places from which the individual can more easily escape. He rubs his genitals against the victim's thighs or buttocks or attempts to fondle breasts. While doing so, he usually fantasizes an exclusive, caring relationship with the victim. Most acts of frottage occur when the person is 15–25 years of age, after which there is general decline in frequency.

As a teenager, Jeffrey Dahmer often fantasized about lying next to a nude male and listening to his heart beat, a desire that fueled his murderous rampage against homosexual males. After strangling his victims, Dahmer often laid next to their corpses to fondle them. Later, he often cannibalized them.

The fantasies, sexual urges, or behaviors cause clinically significant distress or impairment in social, occupational, or in other important areas of functioning. It is designated 302.89 in the DSM.

◼ Sexual Sadism/Sexual Masochism

Alluded to earlier in the section on *Signature Killers,* the sadist involved in **sexual sadism** is characterized by real acts in which the sadist derives sexual excitement from the psychological or physical suffering (including humiliation) of the victim. The fantasies, sexual urges, or behaviors cause clinically significant distress or social or occupational impairment in all perpetrators except for serial offenders. On the other hand, the **masochist** involved in sexual **masochism** involves real acts of being humiliated, beaten, bound, or otherwise made to suffer. The fantasies, sexual urges, or behaviors cause clinically significant distress or social or occupational impairment. Tethered to control and domination, sexual masochism surfaces in a serial killer when his acts humiliate others. Sexual sadism is designated 302.84 and sexual masochism is designated 302.83 in the DSM. **Sadomasochism** combines characteristics of the two paraphilias.

◼ Sexual Disorder NOS

Sexual Disorder NOS (Not Otherwise Specified) is a category for coding a sexual disturbance that does not meet the criteria for any specific sexual disorder and is neither a sexual dysfunction nor a paraphilia. Examples include: marked feelings of inadequacy concerning sexual performance, or other traits related to self-imposed standards of masculinity or femininity; *a succession of lovers who are distressed about repeated sexual relationships experienced by the individual only as things to be used;* persistent and marked distress about sexual orientation.

Individuals with full-blown psychopathic personalities, marked by lack of empathy, have many sexual relationships with people they perceive "as things to be used." The difference between the garden variety psychopath and the sexual psychopath is telling. The sexual psychopath, as a sexual pervert, kills and becomes known to the world as a serial killer—perhaps one of the most perverted such as Ted Bundy.

PREDATOR PROFILE °(4-2)

Theodore "Ted" Bundy

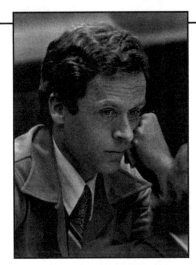
©Bettmann/CORBIS

Media Moniker:

None

Time Span of Crimes:

January 4, 1974–February 9, 1978

Physical Description of Offender:

Normal build, nice looking, white male, dark hair, excellent conversationalist.

Offenses Prior to Serial Killing:

None

Victimology:

Bundy preferred young girls with long brown hair parted down the middle. He acted as if he was hurt and needed help and sympathy from girls he stalked at universities. He brutally raped and murdered his victims.

Current Status:

Executed January 24, 1989, Lethal Injection

General Comments:

Bundy was once an assistant director of the *Seattle Crime Prevention* advisory committee and even wrote a pamphlet instructing women on rape prevention. A one-time Boy Scout with a promising career in Washington state politics, Bundy appeared in the persona of a law student and upstanding citizen. He did charity work and campaigned for the U.S. Republican Party. He grew up in the north end residential area of Tacoma, WA, graduated from the University of Washington and attended the University of Washington Law School. Friends described him as handsome and smart. To girlfriends, he was romantic and tender. To victims, he was a killer; he ripped them apart like a reptile.

     Bundy went on a cross-country murder spree from 1973–1978. State after state, Bundy eluded detection. However, he picked a fistfight with a police officer, who pulled him over on a routine traffic stop while driving a stolen car in Florida in 1978.

Victimology:

1. Joni Lenz, severely beaten in her bed on January 4, 1974. She survived.
2. Lynda Ann Healy, 21, disappeared from her basement bedroom in the University District on February 1, 1974. Healy worked at a radio station.
3. Donna Gail Manson, 19, disappeared from the campus of Evergreen State College on March 12, 1974.
4. Susan Elaine Rancourt, 18, disappeared from the campus of Central Washington State University in Ellensburg on April 17, 1974.
5. Roberta Kathleen Parks, 22, disappeared from the campus of Oregon State University on May 6, 1974.
6. Brenda Carol Ball, 22, last seen in a tavern in Burien on June 1, 1974.
7. Georgann Hawkins, 18, disappeared from behind her sorority house near the University of Washington on June 11, 1974.
8. Janice Ott, 23, and Denise Naslund, 19, both disappeared from Lake Samammish State Park on July 14, 1974.
9. Carol Valenzuela, 20, disappeared near Vancouver, Washington, on August 2, 1974.
10. Laura Aime, 17, disappeared from Lehi, Utah, on October 30, 1974.
11. Nancy Wilcox, 16, a cheerleader, disappeared from Utah in October 1974.
12. Melissa Smith, 17, disappeared from Midvale, Utah, on October 18, 1974.
13. Carol LaRonch, 18, escaped as Bundy tried to kidnap her in Salt Lake City on November 8, 1974.
14. Debby Kent, 17, disappeared from an ice skating rink in Bountiful, Utah, on November 8, 1975.
15. Denise Oliverson, 25, a homemaker, disappeared from Grand Junction, Colorado, April 6, 1975.
16. Connie Cooley, 18, disappeared from Nederland, Colorado, on April 15, 1975.
17. Shelly Robertson, 24, disappeared from Golden, Colorado, on July 1, 1975.
18. Nancy Baird, 23, disappeared from the gas station where she worked in Layton, Utah in 1974.
19. Julie Cunningham, 26, a sporting goods employee, disappeared from Vail, Colorado on March 15, 1975.
20. Caryn Campbell, 23, a nurse, disappeared from the parking lot of her hotel in Utah on January 12, 1975.

SOURCE: *http://www.crimelibrary.com/serial_killers/notorious/index.html*

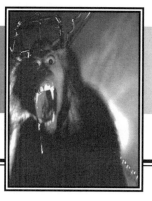

Aftermath

I. Word Scholar

Define the following words from *The Word Scholar Glossary.*

1. Manie sans delire _____

2. Malum in se _____

3. Rape kit _____

4. Successive approximation _____

5. Shaping _____

6. Personation _____

7. Paraphilias _____

8. Overkill _____

9. Staging _____

10. Aftermath _____

II. The Forensic Lab

Compose a one page report addressing the following: Describe the factors in the netherworld—the counterculture of antisocial parenting—you believe are responsible for each stage in developing sexually driven behavior.

CHAPTER 5

The Rapacious Mind: The Neurochemistry of Psychopathy

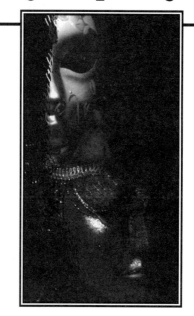

❝You can't reduce me to a set of influences. You've given up good and evil for behaviorism, Officer Starling. You've got everybody in moral dignity pants—nothing is ever anybody's fault. Look at me, Officer Starling. Can you stand to say I'm evil? Am I evil, Officer Starling?"

"I think you're destructive. For me it's the same thing.❞

—*Silence of the Lambs*
Thomas Harris

"There are no crooked thoughts without crooked molecules."

—Sidney Cohen, M.D. (The Chemical Brain)

"I'm not sick, but I'm not well."

—Harvey Danger

A soon to be published book on the criminal psyche, *Guilty by Reason of Insanity,* written by Yale University and Bellevue psychiatrist Dorothy O. Lewis, provides a perfect segue from psychopathic personality of the "mild" to "moderate" garden variety types to conditions in familial milieu that bring about the neurochemical transformation observed in sexual psychopathy. Dr. Lewis, who was the last to interview Ted Bundy before his execution, makes the case that *irreparable neurological damage* plays a significant factor in the mind of serial killers.

■ Perception: A Phenomenological Mix

As we have observed in previous chapters, from the FBI model of criminal profiling to current modifications in North America and Europe, the *art and science* of profiling serial killers rests solidly upon the behavioral sciences. In this chapter, we add the contributions of *neuropsychology*—the interdisciplinary biological, neurological, and psychological specialty—that studies powerful neurotransmitters and neurohormones and how powerful chemical "cocktails" of circulating chemistry "rewire" cortices in the brain. **Nature** (neurochemistry) and **nurture** (social learning) set up powerful cognitive maps of learning, comprising an individual's **phenomenological** perception of the world. It explains how we "interpret" others, how we relate to them, and what we expect. This internal sense (not unlike our internal "sense of self") is influential across a wide continuum of behavior.

As a behavioral science, psychology studies *behavior across a continuum,* a line suggesting possibilities. With psychopathy as our subject, let's label the midpoint of the continuum "normal"; to the far right "psychotic," and to the far left "criminally abnormal". Sexual psychopathy is not psychotic behavior, therefore, on the continuum it belongs to the far left under "criminally abnormal". (Recall Pinel's *manie dans delire.*) The brain of sexual psychopaths has been substantially changed (enough we think to warrant the label Homo pseudo-sapient.)

According to **cognitive neuroscience**, *experiences* merge with neurochemistry to produce cognitive "scripts" that direct behavior and expectations with chemical underpinnings. Chemical "cocktails" of circulating neurochemistry provide the **pluripotent** emotional foundations between *affective* ("feeling") states and *cognitive* ("thinking") residing deep within the brain's pleasure pathways.

It is in the brain—deep in neural tissue—that we become scholars, saints, or sadists, the inner sanctum of sanctified minds, intellectual minds, and rapacious minds.

■ Postpartum Growth

Speculation varies, but many brain researchers believe over 70% of the human brain develops after birth. Therefore, developmental glitches from a variety of abuses—verbal, physical, sexual, as well as emotional neglect, and the everyday stress and tension inherent in coping with antisocial parenting—"rewires" the brain of sexual predators in deleterious ways we are just beginning to understand.

As we have seen, mental health professionals agree a major contributor to *rapacious behavior* observed in sexual psychopathy is the abuse dictated upon children from hateful antisocial parenting, and the concomitant lack of *life-affirming experiences of affection and bonding* to family members. Studies by Harlow, Bowlby, and others, suggest developmental scarcities or physical trauma (being slapped, hit, or slugged in the head) rewire the brain in permanent ways before age two. The effect of *cumulative trauma* "presents" as "cool-coded" brain scans observed in sexual psychopaths. This type of trauma is the neurological damage suggested by Lewis in her book.

■ Emotional Rootedness

It is not surprising that those who "slowly simmer" developmentally as sexual psychopaths, and soon-to-be serial predators, don't experience emotional bonding or what the 1970's developmental psychologists called emotional **rootedness**. They don't feel loved. They don't feel valued. They feel depersonalized. To compensate, they try to inflate their own self-importance. Like the alcoholic and drug addict, everything revolves in their own orbit. The organized serial killer's attitude is often marked by egotism, narcissism, and arrogance. To the psychopath, he's been denied his rightful place at the banquet table of life. While many children overcome and rise above "bad parenting"—*incompetent, absent, and/or minimally skilled parenting* to become successful and productive citizens, few, if any, rise about horrific antisocial parenting.

We will identify in this chapter "the one indispensable ingredient"— the final stake in the heart in the developing sexual psychopath that ends in serial killing, after an overview of neurochemical underpinnings of psychopathy.

■ *Manie Sans Delire*

As previously mentioned a theme that runs throughout this book, forensic neuropsychologists and psychiatrists find that most serial predators are not psychotic. Recall Pinel's term *manie sans delire*—"obsession without insanity." Criminal psychopaths, although neurologically damaged, *know exactly what they're doing*. Most are not paranoid schizophrenics, although some were (e.g. David Berkowitz and Richard Trenton Chase). For serial predators, normal chemistry becomes maligned, and ultimately, rapacious, due in great part to what we present in this chapter.

This chapter goes beyond the superficial personas of criminal predators down to the tissue level of human behavior, personality, and ultimately, the *feelings*—the burning torch that drives serial rapacity. Make no mistake about it, serial rapists and killers rape and murder victims because of the way it makes them *feel*. They "feel" their way from crime to crime like a reptile "feels" with his tongue.

Due to hateful antisocial parenting, directly resulting in severe glitches in normal brain development, the "becoming" sexual psychopath is *emotionally retarded,* yet 100% sure what makes him feel good—sexually preying upon victims. If he experiences self-hatred the next day for his rapacious behavior, he finds ways to **rationalize**, **intellectualize**, or **deny** the brutality of it, just like the alcoholic denies his vociferous addiction. Soon, killers feels the sexualized "brutal urge" welling up inside of them again as though a dose of Viagra® kicked in. He is ready to destroy his next victim.

■ Perception

As mentioned earlier, **perception** is the key to "processing" reality. When the comedic actor Gene Wilder (in the movie *Young Frankenstein*) discovered his loyal lab assistant Igor had stolen a beaker from the medical school containing a brain labeled "Abby Normal" he had just transplanted into Frankenstein's monster, he knew the world was in big trouble. The monster's abnormal ("Abby Normal") brain could never experience or process reality in normal ways. Alas, the creature was destined to be a creature, a *Homo pseudo-sapien.*

Using documented research (as inductive logic) and speculative reasoning (as deductive logic), we will identify the chemical messengers that kindle the unrelenting feelings within the mind of normal, everyday individuals, as well as how the same chemistry "turns" rapacious and produces pseudo-sapient creatures.

■ Brain: Absolute Monarch of Behavior

What drives cognitive and affective states of human behavior, observed across a behavioral continuum that is both wide and long, stretching between normalcy and insanity? To the **neuroscientist**, the answer is deceptively simple, yet justifiably complex: the answer is the brain—the organ of behavior, and its powerful battalion of neurochemistry and hormones.

Normalcy, dysfunction, psychopathy, and **addiction** are under the sole jurisdiction of the brain and its chemical messengers and neurohormones of the body. Addiction—whether to drugs, raping, or killing, is more about *feeling* than about thinking. Yet, as *Alcoholics Anonymous (AA)* proclaim, "addicts must deal with "stinking thinking". Regardless, *the brain is the absolute monarch of behavior, thinking, and feeling.*

Normal and abnormal behaving individuals continue to do what makes them *feel the way they want to feel,* from the successful entrepreneur to the raging alcoholic to the sexual predator. *It's all about feeling:* "no crooked thoughts without crooked molecules". For the serial killer: "no rapacious thoughts without the chemistry that produces rapacious behavior.

Addiction has receptors deep in the brain, down in the **reptilian brain** of the brain stem, and further up in the limbic system's "pleasure pathways" within a neural structure known as the **MFB (medial forebrain bundle)**. The chemistry of pleasure, mediated by **dopamine (DA)**, and to some extent **norepinephrine (NE)** and other chemistry covered in the section, justifies feeling **hedonistic**, ultimately explaining why individuals become addicted to everything from apple pie to serial killing.

■ The Addict's Pacifier—Addiction to "Jazzed" Chemistry

At the core of normalcy, dysfunction, criminality, and the deviant psyches of serial killers lies the answer—the brain's ability of *self-addiction,* whereby individuals become addicted to their own neurochemistry. "Rewiring" neural tissue in the direction of sexual psychopathy occurs due to a steady "diet" of persistent dysfunctional learning, deviant fantasies, and developmental glitches retarding normal brain development. Since the brain thrives by "sprouting" new axons and pairing back old ones, new "connections" emanating from the mind of sexual psychopaths reinforce what drives axonal development, that is, the propensity for perverted sexual *thinking,* not normal, rational thinking.

■ Holistic Nature of Brain-Mind-Body

Neuroscientists analyze human behavior without regard to the ancient dichotomy of mind-body dualism. **Dualism** states that mind is a separate entity (mentalistic), while body is another (physical). Therefore, there will always be discrepancies in analyzing behavior because the two entities—mental versus physical—cannot be blended into one compatible entity. The old, pre-scientific argument maintained brain-mind-body produced a hopeless conundrum. Not anymore.

Modern neuroscientists adhere to the **holistic** theory of the integration of brain-mind-body. In this perspective, the skin acts as a kind of outermost covering of the brain since neural components influence each other to varying degrees. Interestingly, the behaviorists were the first to argue the notion of "whole body" orientation. For example, a pregnant women is pregnant "through and through"—in her mind, body, and brain—not just her belly. Sadly, so are sexual predators.

In this holistic brain-body configuration, the body is the "action figure"—glands and hormones, (the "blood messengers"), muscles, (the "prime movers"), and neurotransmitters (the emotional "thermostat" for circulating chemistry). The outpouring of feeling, mood, thinking, and behavior characterizes what cognitive neuroscientists observe as "mind" or "personality."

The argument that some drugs (such as marijuana and its addictive agent *cannabis sativa*) may be *psychologically* addictive, but not *physiologically* addictive, ignores the holistic nature of brain-body. The point is: if an addict doesn't smoke "weed" for a while, he's going to crave it. What difference does it make whether or not it's from brain, body, or mind. The addict craves the feeling, regardless of the source. The following analogy will help those still doubtful of brain-body holism. When separately felt by a blind person, the tusk, ears, and truck of an elephant feel like they don't belong on the same animal, yet, they comprise the totality of what the world knows as "elephant", regardless of separate part. By the same token, we are not separate parts. It's time to leave the "part and parcel" thinking of the 1970's behind and move forward into the holistic view of the twenty-first century of neuroscience.

■ Connectivity

The spinal cord connects the CNS (**central nervous system**)—brain and spinal cord—to the body, housing the PNS (**peripheral nervous system**).

This confluence of brain-body sets up the concept of "mind"—the perfect metaphor for this union —as the *mental component.*

What causes normal chemistry to be *transformed into macabre and rapacious perversion* so prevalent in serial crime?

The brain-body of serial rapists and murderers "house" the same chemistry cascading in the pleasure pathways of the MFB as normal individuals. However, due to *deviant cognitive maps,* perverted sexual thinking and fantasy results. With countless neurons screaming for dopamine and other pleasurable chemistry that lies behind the "thrilling high" caused by the addiction to perverted fantasy, the motivation is "compelling" and overwhelming. Cognitively, the domain of restraint is muted. (The Reagan Administration's failed drug message: "Just say no"! shows the ignorance of politicians regarding the power of brain chemistry.)

■ Habituation versus Addiction

The 2.5-pound human brain with the consistency of hard Jell-O® is unsurpassed in the universe for complexity of connectivity, organization, function, and chemical configuration. Working together as chemical precursors to all behavior, feeling, thinking, and mood, the brain-body's neurochemistry explains why brain-body-mind can be understood in chemical terms with habituation (learned habits) at one end of the behavioral continuum and addiction at the other.

Suddenly, we see how easily we pick up habits and keep them. If our habits produce "jazzed feelings" (due to brain chemistry), we usually keep them; however, if they produce uncomfortable or negative feelings (again due to brain chemistry), we usually modify or drop them like . . . well . . . like a bad habit, unless, of course, addiction enters the picture. Addiction changes everything.

Edward L. Thorndike's *Law of Effect* and John B. Watson's *S→R psychology* proved how habits are purely behavioral by famous experiments. To the behaviorist, we learn, communicate, live in families, relax with friends, do our jobs, engage in sex, and create art, literature, and science due to habituation—habitual behavior. Idiomatically, we are truly "creatures of habit." In functional and competent milieus we become socialized as responsible, productive, and achievement-oriented individuals. Goal-driven behavior is possible through our "higher order" cognitive skills due to generous twin cerebral hemispheres and the overlay of neocortex (literally, "new bark"). Proactive and goal-directed thinking seems to provide "tracks" for neurochemistry and hormones to dispense feeling to "run" upon.

■ Addiction—Habituation Takes a Deadly Turn

However, when an individual becomes addicted to a powerful aphrodisiac-like mix of his own neurochemistry, he feels *compelled* to continue whatever activity produced the feeling, even though the addict knows the activity is harmful or criminal. Addiction works that way. Addiction to hardcore pornography may start as habituation; viewing "porn" a few times a month can lead some individuals to an obsessive-compulsive addiction so that watching it continually day after day becomes a "brutal urge." In the process, the viewer becomes a *slave to his own biochemistry*. Just like the **sex addict** who is addicted to the feeling produced by the physical act of sex in the pleasure pathways of the brain, he continues to seek sex for the feeling it gives him. The same scenario is true for the "crank" addict who is hopelessly addicted to methamphetamine, where only 6% of "crank" addicts fully recover; that's 94% who don't. Residing in close proximity to this number, 0% of sexual predators recover.

Interestingly, ritualistic, obsessive, compulsive, and sexualized behavior characterizes addiction. Neural receptors deep in the brain facilitate the process of addiction.

Can addiction turn addicts away from "higher order" thinking, characteristic of neural centers in the cerebrum, prefrontal lobes, and neocortex—areas characterized by behavioral restraint and consideration of consequences? Does *addiction* to the "thrilling highs" of pleasurable chemistry reside in a completely different area than the "higher order" centers so prevalent in civilized human behavior?

Researchers such as Paul MacLean point to the lower, pre-verbal, **reptilian brain** as a source. Presently, the reptilian brain theory of serial predators will be presented with compelling arguments that psychopathy may reside in this ancient structure present in humans as well as reptiles.

In the process of delineating the cyto-architecture of the brain, we will make a systematic attempt to apply what neuroscience has discovered in painstaking research regarding powerful neurotransmitters, **second messenger peptides**, and neurohormones known to underlie normal, as well as abnormal and criminal behavior.

When "higher-order" brain centers in the cerebrum, prefrontal lobes, and neocortex are underdeveloped or traumatized due to physical, sexual, or verbal abuse from antisocial parenting, there is the possibility that primitive *reptilian centers* in the brainstem exert powerful influences over focus and motivation in life. It is true the serial predator perceives such a different world than a normal person with normal brain development. The serial killer and cannibal Jeffery Dahmer, provides an example.

PREDATOR PROFILE (5-1)

Jeffrey Lionel Dahmer
"The Milwaukee Cannibal"

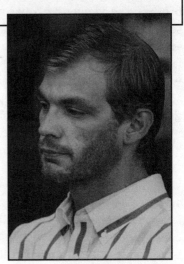

©Reuters Newmedia Inc./CORBIS

Time Span of Crimes:

1978–1991

Physical Description:

White male in his mid-30s, thin body, brown hair, brown eyes

Born:

May 21st, 1960 in Milwaukee.

Current Status:

Deceased (killed in prison)

Prior Offenses:

Sexual Assault, public intoxication.

Victimology:

Dahmer's victims were young males ages 14–32. Most of the victims were black or Hispanic gay men. Excluding his first victim, all victims were picked up at bars or grocery stores, promised sex, drugs, alcohol, or pornography back at his apartment.

Jeffrey drugged and experimented with the live victims, then strangled, dismembered, eviscerated, and committed necrophilia on the victims.

Dahmer preserved some parts of the victims' bodies and cannibalized them in some cases. He always strangled his victims, claiming it was the least painful way he could think of killing them. He also took many photos which he archived in a macabre "gallery of death" photo album.

Childhood of a Monster

Jeffrey Lionel Dahmer was born in Wisconsin in 1960. His family moved often during the early years of his life. Dahmer's parents were unhappily married and spent most of their time fighting with one another. Dahmer had one younger brother named David.

From the beginning, Dahmer had medical problems. He was born with broken legs and had to wear splints until he was three years old. He couldn't walk until he was two and had to have help standing up. At the age of four, he had surgery for a hernia. He recalled the experience as "embarrassing." He was in intense pain. At one point, he thought the doctors had cut off his penis. He felt emotionally scarred from this event. As he grew up he was quiet and kept to himself. At the age of eight, it was rumored a neighbor boy molested him although nothing was proven. Soon after this incident, Dahmer became introverted and disruptive. He made a spectacle of himself in class as the class clown. He was considered to be a bright child by his teachers, but only managed average grades.

As an adolescent, Dahmer experimented with the dead carcasses of animals. This macabre event coincided with the start of puberty. He brought road kill home and clandestinely performed autopsies on them. Since his father was a chemist, Dahmer used his knowledge of acids to dissolve tissue from the bone. He began to fantasize what humans would look like "on the inside." Dahmer was discovering that along with puberty he was becoming attracted to men. He didn't know how to handle this urge so he began to drink in an effort to self-medicate. He was plagued by the fantasy of lying next to an unconscious person, someone who could meet his needs, but would not ask anything in return.

Dahmer became an alcoholic, attempting to suppress his disturbing thoughts but eventually, he was compelled to act out and murder his first victim. Dahmer hid in the woods one day hoping to disable a male jogger who frequently ran along the path. He took a baseball bat and planned to knock him into unconsciousness and just lie down next to him. Luckily, the jogger didn't come by that day and Dahmer went home.

Dahmer's parents divorced when he turned 18 years of age. His mother received custody of Jeff and his brother David. Soon after, however, his mother and David abandoned him, leaving Jeff home alone. He called his father, who eventually moved back into the family home with him. However, his father would soon leave him too. This time, Dahmer moved in with his grandmother and soon sought out his first victim.

Victimology

Dahmer's first victim was hitchhiker Stephen Hicks. He talked Hicks into coming back to his place to get drunk. After having a few beers, Dahmer beat Hicks to death. Dahmer threw the body in a crawl space under his house.

A few days later, he dismembered the corpse and burned the tissue off the bones, then ground the bones into dust and spread them in his backyard. Dahmer never intended to commit another crime.

Eventually his grandmother asked Dahmer to leave her house because of foul smells coming from his room. Dahmer joined the army and became a field medic, where he learned more about human anatomy. When he left the army, he rented an apartment in Milwaukee, Wisconsin. This is where many grisly murders took place nine years later.

Dahmer was almost caught twice by policemen. The first time occurred during his first murder when he was pulled over for drunk driving. He had Stephen Hick's body in the backseat in a bag. The cop let him go without checking the bag. The second time occurred when a 14-year-old naked boy escaped Dahmer's apartment drugged and incoherent. Two young black girls witnessing the event called police. The police arrived and sent the boy back to Dahmer's apartment as Dahmer claimed they were lovers and got into a fight. Dahmer then butchered the boy.

A Violent Ending

Dahmer was caught in 1991. To the shock and horror of authorities his apartment contained many human body parts, lying out in the open and in his refrigerator. They also found a 55-gallon drum in which he stored acid to dispose of torsos and unwanted body parts.

At trial, Dahmer was declared sane and sentenced to 957 consecutive years in prison, since Wisconsin has no death penalty. In 1994, a black male inmate beat him to death.

◨ The Reptilian "Processor"

Strong evidence exists from brain scanning technology that the reptilian brain (and the mid-brain and amygdala) take center stage as the "processor" of reality for serial killers (sexual psychopaths) instead of "higher-order" centers of reason, appropriateness, and restraint observed in the cerebrum, neocortex, and normalized prefrontal lobes. It appears that in psychopathy, electrochemical "signals" are not "broadcast" appropriately in the underdeveloped "higher-order" centers. Restraint and social appropriateness, so conspicuously absent from sexual psychopaths, cannot compete with the more visceral aspects of reptilian "lower centers." If this were not so, why does the rapacious behavior of serial predators remind investigators of wild animal attacks on victims where vicious rape and mutilation ("overkill") is such a common occurrence? The brutality of some crime scenes suggests an animal attacked the victim. How could a Homo sapien (a human being with thinking and reason) be responsible for such staggering violence?

◨ The Reptilian Brain: Theory & Implications

When all of the regalia of societal camouflage is removed from sexual psychopaths so that social *persona* afforded by clothes, social roles, job title, campus identity (if any), conversational "gift of gab," and impersonation (such as clowns, handymen, or police officers) are stripped away, what's left is little more than *a reptile with reptilian appetites* hiding behind a human face.

Characterized by a "big swelling" at the top of the spinal cord, the reptilian brain is the oldest, most primitive part of our *gray matter* (dominated by **myelinized** axons). The **brain stem** and **cerebellum** comprise the reptilian brain.

◨ The Brain Stem

The **brain stem** is composed of the medulla, pons, cerebellum, the mesencephalon—comprising the red nucleus and the substantia nigra—globus pallidus, olfactory bulbs, and the basal nuclei.

1. The complete name of the *medulla* is the **medulla oblongata** and in brain anatomy termed **myelencephalon**. It is located at the most *caudal* (tail-end) point of the brain stem and fuses with the spinal cord at the skull. It is responsible for *autonomic* (autonomic) functions of heart rate, respiration, and blood pressure. Additional nuclei belong to the **RAS** (reticular activation system) of the brain stem where activity from the senses is integrated into attention, arousal, and mediation of sleep-wake states. In sexual psychopathy, a convincing argument exists that the **thalamus** produces *a low "amplification"* of incoming sensory data

that normally broadcasts to higher centers. Due to the weak "broadcast," *craving more stimulation* may occur. In a normal brain, a similar condition (without pathology) characterizes the so-called *extravert*—a "people person" who craves stimulation from others. In a neurologically damaged brain, the person acts out with a *rapacious mind,* intent upon raping and murdering others to experience and re-experience the "thrilling high." (In contrast, so-called high "amplification" from the thalamus in normal individuals results in attempts to *reduce stimulation* observed in so-called "introverts" who do not require social opportunities of high stimulation). The medulla is the only brain structure linking *higher brain centers with spinal cord* functioning.

2. *The Pons and the Cerebellum.* The pons and the cerebellum comprise the **metencephalon.** The *dorsal (toward the back) aspect of the pons* is the **pontine tegmentum,** which "broadcasts" powerful neurotransmitter activity into various regions of the nervous system including *serotonin* (5-HT). When 5-HT is liberated at the synapse, it leads to the well documented "4-Cs of feeling"—calm, cool, collected, and confident. However, when this powerful neurotransmitter is blocked by other regulating chemistry, the scarcity of 5-HT leads to feeling "empty," depressed, or emotionally unsettled. Another chemical with ubiquitous "broadcast" is referred to as an "adrenergic" transmitter, characterized by *norepinephrine* (NE) and *adrenaline* "working" (hence "ergic") leading to feeling "jazzed," focused, and interested. When blocked, a scarcity of NE (and adrenaline) leads to lack of motivation and muted interest in almost everything. Finally, *acetylcholine* (Ach)— the ubiquitous parasympathetic chemical "calmer" lying behind a multitude of behavior, including sexuality, is the third ubiquitously "broadcast" chemical. The **cerebellum** (literally, "small brain") controls and stabilizes movements, coordination, and muscle tone. As observed in both the Bowlby and Harlow studies of "contact comfort," social bonding, and motion, deficits in cerebellar function can have impoverished effects upon "higher-order" behavior, across a wide spectrum.

3. *Mesencephalon.* The **mesencephalon** is comprised of the red nucleus and **substantia nigra** (black substance). *Control of movement* is the function of the red nucleus, while the substantia nigra has two nuclei rich in dopamine (DA)—the neurotransmitter behind pleasure. When this region looses a substantial amount of receptors, the movement disorder Parkinsonism is diagnosed.

4. *Globus Pallidus.* Known as the paleostriatum—"old striatum"—it is one of four basal ganglia composed of gray matter within each cerebral hemisphere involved in the control of movement.

5. *Olfactory Bulbs.* Sensory center for the detection of smell and odors.

The brain stem is innervated with neurons that provide *basic emotions* such as fear, lust, love, and hate. It is the center of *aggression* and the *motivation for survival.*

In this vital brain area, *the brain of humans shares the same behavioral agenda as snakes and lizards.* Therefore, we contend that a human, whose rapacious behavior stems in great measure from the reptilian brain, should be reclassified in sub-human terms as a *pseudo-sapien.*

Similar to a needle being stuck in the groove of an old 45-RPM record, the brainstem houses neural structures that are *highly repetitious and ritualistic,* producing behavior that is obsessive-compulsive and **paranoid**, never learning from prior behavior. The brainstem remains active in deep sleep.

Millions of years of brain evolution have added layers upon layers of soft tissue in the *cerebral cortexes* and **neocortex** (literally "new bark")—the thin layer of recently evolved tissue covering the brain like a micro-thin cap. Along with the **frontal lobes**, these "higher order" centers promote *complex thinking abilities* such as reasoning, strategizing, decision-making, and intellectual curiosity. Consequences—pro and con—for behavior choices reside in these centers.

Like Freud's metaphorical id, the reptilian brain "operates" as if seeking pleasure (and avoiding pain), feeding, and foraging. This ancient blueprint for survival is *impatient and activity-oriented.* It lies behind the emotional mania of success at whatever cost. It provides the energy behind the idiom "success breeds success" or the scary inner world of hedonistic appetites. For survival, it has a "search and destroy" mentality.

In short, we propose strong empirical evidence from neuroimaging of the brain provides compelling speculative logic that the *reptilian brain lies behind rapacious behavior especially when other cortices, such as the cerebellum and prefrontal lobes, have been traumatized.*

■ Dreams Crushed

When viewing the A & E produced taped interview of convicted serial killer Ted Bundy moderated by Dr. James Dobson, Ph.D., the camera targets a close up of Bundy's face on numerous occasions. Not much imagination is required to perceive Bundy's facial demeanor, especially his mouth, resembling a lizard!

Can years of antisocial parenting producing rapacious behavior result in the very likeness of a reptile?

When lifelong dreams are crushed, violence is unleashed in some individuals with severe neurological damage to cortices in their brain. A percentage of such individuals will lash out in anger or rage in retaliation for being denied. Charles Manson sought stardom as a rock singer; Ted Bundy sought a law degree; Wayne Williams felt destined to become a police officer; Adolph Hitler sought to become an famous artist and so the list goes on. They were all crushed by failure. Eventually failing multiple suicide attempts (in some instances), they acted out violently as rapists, murderers, or mass murderers. No single root cause exists to explain the Mansons, the Bundys, or the Hiltlers. No single root cause exits because there is none. But, a lethal combination of horrific experiences and the accommodation of neurochemistry, along with a "triggering" event, can.

According to proponents of the reptilian brain theory, this region "powers" artists as well as murderers. Non-judgmental, it possesses no independent cognition to distinguish between right and wrong; it wants activity—any activity. At time it can be impulsive, at other times compulsive. **Obsessive-compulsive disorder (OCD)**, **Post-Traumatic Stress Disorder (PTSD)**, and **panic disorder** are presumed to occur in reptilian cortical "processors."

Add the androgenic hormone **testosterone** to "fuel" the passion of emotional behavior and it is suddenly understandable, perhaps even logical, why very young individuals in their twenties to mid-thirties age group are so driven—driven to achieve, or in the alternative, driven to destroy. This age span and the precursor teenage years (from ages 12 to 18) produce the most distinguishable age group of great achievement (young actors, directors, writers, inventors, artists, scholars, soldiers, and athletes). Those who seek to achieve socially approved goals reside at one end of the continuum—the "creators"—while serial killers and other criminals "infest" the other end—as "destroyers."

In fact, in the non-criminal sense, it is normal for young adolescent males (ages 16 to 19) and young adult males (about 20 to 35 years of age) to be serial, sexual "predators". In a normal sense, most males in these age categories are on the prowl to "score" as much sex as possible—not in the mode of a killer or rapist—but as a **lothario** or sexual Don Juan, who experiences a variety of sexual partners. Studies show that most males experience the most sexual activity of their lives at this time and age group. It is not too far-fetched to propose individuals who become sexual psychopaths are out of control with sexualized rage, anger, or revenge where the reptilian brain overrides "higher order" rational brain components.

An alternative explanation exists. If chemical signals are so weak in the brain stem and "midbrain" relating to feeling pleasure, psychopaths may seek *extreme measures,* such as rape and murder, in an attempt to feel any pleasure at all. Although speculative, this theory cannot be ignored.

◾ The Limbic System

The "mid-brain" residing just above the reptilian brain and below the twin "cams" of the cerebrum corresponds to the brain of most mammals, such as dogs and cats. Termed "old mammalian brain," it adds another layer of cerebral tissue to mental and emotional capabilities. According to researcher Paul MacLean, who coined the term *limbic system* in 1952 (coincidently, the same year REM research began), the "middle brain" is concerned with "emotions and instincts, feeding, fleeing, fighting, and sexual behavior".

MacLean maintains everything in this *emotional center* is either "agreeable or disagreeable"; survival depends on avoidance of pain and repetition of pleasure. According to MacLean the limbic system determines "*valence*—whether or not we feel *positive or negative* about something" and "*salience*—what gets our attention." It has *extensive connections* to the "higher" brain, the neocortex. The limbic system contains the following neural structures: hypothalamus, hippocampus, and amygdala.

1. The **hypothalamus** is the blood-chemistry monitor of the CNS and a primary organizer of the cascading endocrine system of hormones produced by ductless glands sending hormones to remote binding sites within the body-brain. The *medial forebrain bundle* is located within the neural tissue of the hypothalamus.

2. The **hippocampus** is the center for learning and memory.
3. The **amygdala** is the center for emotional memory and aggression. Recent research implicates this region in violent behavior.

◼ Lesch-Nyhan Syndrome (LNS)

In **Lesch-Nyhan Syndrome** (lesh-neye-en), perhaps no better example exists for the role of the midbrain and neurochemistry in so-called "primitive behavior"—such as aggression, feeding, and rapacious (preying) behavior. Lesch-Nyhan syndrome (LNS) is an extremely rare *genetic mutation of the X chromosome* in boys, occurring in approximately one in one million births. Lesch-Nyhan boys lack *one* enzyme, hypoxanthine-guanine phosphoribosyltransferase (HPRT), resulting in an excess of uric acid in the bloodstream. Early symptoms include uric acid crystals passed from the kidneys appearing as "orange sand" in the diapers.

By age one, physical symptoms become predominant as normal coordination is replaced by full body spasticity and rigidity in the limbs. His body position appears in the characteristic "fencing" posture—one arm bent with the opposite leg bent—evidence of neurological damage to the midbrain. In childhood, as he gets stronger, *he becomes an unwilling predator* to himself in self-mutilating behavior and to others, even those he loves. He attacks with his teeth. He tries to pull out his own fingernails with his teeth. He may eat his own fingers. Some Lesch-Nyhan boys have lost most of their own lips due to autocannibalism. Like the brain damaged sexual psychopath, *they know what they're doing but they can't stop.* They have no choice; they feel compelled to continue ritualistic self-mutilating behavior.

In one of the most startling characteristics of LNS, they may rip their own eyes out of the sockets in self-enucleation. When they feel an episode of self-mutilation coming on they beg to have their body restrained. Reaching adulthood is rare. The prognosis for boys with LNS is poor. Like sexual psychopaths, there is no treatment. The neurological defects are irreversible. The abnormal build-up of uric acid within the body causes the agonizing episodes of self-mutilation and ultimately death due to kidney failure or self-injury.

The neurological damage of LNS, so starkly evident in posturing and behavior (spasticity, rigidity, the "fencing" posture, and biting), is absent in sexual psychopathy (except for biting for sexual gratification). Yet, like LNS boys, they have damaged midbrains—the seat of aggression and rapacity. They most certainly have damaged prefrontal lobes—"behavioral brakes", now muted by irreversible neurological damage, allowing full expression of midbrain rapacity. In severe cases, damage to temporal lobes, amygdala, and cerebellum are noted in sexual psychopathy.

Because the appearance and behavior of (organized) sexual psychopaths appear normal, *feeling safe is the danger* in the presence of a reptile hiding behind a human face; the severity of his neurological damage so well disguised in a normal body. The devastation of rapacious behavior left behind in the wake of serial homicide is the only hint of his rapacious psychopathy and explains why he is so very dangerous to others. He is the ultimate paradox of appearing human on the surface, yet willingly preying upon others as a reptile. No one sees him coming.

■ The Higher Echelon Brain— The Neocortex

The most recently developed brain tissue consists of the twin hemispheres of the cerebrum, and the upper-most thin layer of cells called the *neocortex* ("new bark"). The neocortex is responsible for higher cognitive functions such as *cognitive strategies,* complex social interactions, and advanced planning. MacLean refers to this area as "the mother of invention and the father of abstract thought." The left and right hemispheres of the cerebrum take up the major portion of total brain mass. The right side of the cerebrum specializes in "artistic and musical proclivities, spatial and abstract thought," while the left side is more "linear, rational and verbal."

■ Cognitive Neuroscience— The Association Cortices

One of the most intriguing aspects of the human brain is its ability to generate thoughts and feelings, allowing humans to learn and express feelings so effortlessly in both *body language* and *verbal language.* Since everyday interaction as well as the creation of culture and its continuance depends upon *complex mental functions,* scientists are slowly deciphering the structural and functional organization of relevant brain regions. In the booming field of medical technology, the development of *noninvasive brain imaging* as well as complimentary animal studies in nonhuman primates are disclosing "cellular correlates" in specific brain areas to observable behavior. *Cognitive neuroscience* is the term most often used to describe this rapidly growing body of knowledge.

The diverse functions of the **association cortices** of the human brain are loosely referred to as *cognition*—the process by which we come to know and perceive the world. The association cortices integrate information from a variety of sources—*inputs* to the cortices include projections from sensory and motor cortices, the thalamus, and "lower centers" in the brain stem. *Outputs* from the association cortices reach the hippocampus, basal ganglia, cerebellum, and thalamus.

Neuroscientists understand the role of the cortices and connections from the following sources: neurological patients, functional mapping of the brain during neurosurgery, animal studies, and brain scanning technology such as Positron Emission Tomography (PET), Brain Electrical Activity Mapping (BEAM), and Superconducting Interference Device (SQUID). Using these diverse sources, cognitive neuroscientists believe the human ability of attending, identifying, and planning appropriate behavior occurs in the following *association cortices:*

1. The *parietal* association cortex is important for *attending* to complex stimuli in the external and internal environment,
2. The *temporal* association cortex is important in *identifying* the nature of such stimuli, and
3. The *frontal* association cortex is important in *planning* appropriate behavioral responses to the stimuli.

The association cortices of the parietal, temporal, and frontal lobes make cognition possible.

◼ Prefrontal Lobe Damage—The Case of Phines Gage

Being the largest lobe with the most *diverse repertoire of functions*, deficits resulting from damage to the *prefrontal lobes* are devastating. Behavioral deficits observed after frontal lobe damage reflects what we normally describe as an individual's "personality" or "self-in-relation-to-the-world". The case that first brought attention to this connection was prefrontal lobe damage to Phines Gage, a railroad worker in the mid-1850s. A vociferous explosion changed his character or personality forever. Accidentally, a heavy metal rod was driven through his left eye socket destroying most of the prefrontal lobe. Miraculously, Gage recovered physically. His outward appearance appeared normal. However, to his coworkers, Gage was never the "same person."

Subsequent to the accident, the once hard-working foreman, universally respected by his peers, had become "an inconsiderate, intemperate lout". Regarding his abrupt change in character, a physician wrote,

> ". . . his mind was radically changed . . . (into) . . . a child in intellectual capacity . . . he has the animal passions of a strong man . . . he was no longer 'Gage' ".

Another patient followed by neurologists in the 1920s–1930s, lost most of both prefrontal lobes to a fast spreading neoplasm (tumor). Although he retained a high degree of intellectual functioning, his personality changed. He became "boastful of his professional, physical, and sexual prowess . . . showing *little restraint and appropriateness.*"

◼ Lobotomy, Concussion, and Contusion

In a related way, the thousands of *frontal lobotomies* performed in the 1930s–1940s as a primitive form of "neurosurgery" document further the change of personality or character following prefrontal lobe damage. Prefrontal lobe damage does not have to be due to injury by a steel rod or lobotomy. "Rewiring" can occur due to severe parental abuses, physical strikes to the head and other neurological injuries observed in **shaken baby syndrome** and variations such as **concussion** or **contusion** where association cortices are irreversibly damaged.

Clinicians note that some of the most debilitating psychiatric disorders involve the emotions. Neuroscientists know that emotional expression is closely tied to the visceral motor system—the *autonomic nervous system (ANS)* and the *somatic motor system,* especially evidenced in facial muscles and central brain structures governing preganglionic neurons in the brainstem and spinal cord. Other key brain areas in emotional processing are the limbic system, amygdala, and prefrontal lobes.

Experimental psychologist Philip Bard (1928) showed that the *hypothalamus* is a critical area for coordination of emotional behavior in a series of experiments in cats involving duel **hemispherectomy**. With both cerebral hemispheres (including cortex and basal ganglia) removed, the cats subsequently acted enraged. Bard labeled the behavior "sham rage" because it had no obvious target. It's not a big leap to suggest damage to these areas in humans, due to the emotional fallout from hateful antisocial parenting, can produce rage.

Referencing information obtained from association cortices and the aforementioned brain scanners, violent criminals have shown impairment in the prefrontal lobes, thalamus, medial temporal lobe, and left angular gyrus. According to Siegel (2003), a review of the literature and research by Nathaniel Palone and James Hennessy find that chronic violent criminals have higher levels of brain dysfunction than the general population; in the case of homicide offenders—those who kill—it is *32 times greater.*

■ The Brains of Sexual Psychopaths— Born or Made?

A disturbing statistic is that approximately 20% of maximum-security prison population is composed of garden variety psychopaths who are responsible for *over half* the crimes committed. Since "white collar" criminals and drug laundering comprise a large number of inmates in a minimum-security prison, the number of incarcerated psychopaths may treble the number of maximum-security inmates. In white collar crimes, "mild" to "moderate" psychopaths (not sexual psychopaths) are responsible for 80–90% of the crimes.

According to British researchers, garden variety psychopaths do not experience normal emotions such as love, emotional connection or empathy. They do not experience "vibes" for other people like normal individuals. Simply, they just don't care about people *except for sexual stimulation.* Period. According to a study in the UK, one in every 200 citizens is garden variety psychopath. The majority of psychopaths are not in prison for violent acts. However, the range of their crimes makes them Public Enemy #1. Some simply vanish; they abandon girlfriends, family, and jobs; they move from state to state just like they move from person to person.

■ Looking Beyond Words

Who are the non-criminal psychopaths? According to Robert Hare, who has spent over twenty-five years studying "the psychopath" and knows more about psychopathy than anyone else in the world, his *Psychopathic Checklist* provides clues. A score of 26 or higher (out of a possible score of 40) indicates psychopathy. That psychopaths display engaging personalities and a "gift of gab" is one of the biggest surprises to those unfamiliar with the chameleon aspects of their charming and persona-driven personality.

Recognizing psychopathy means *to look beyond his words . . . look for irrationality and excessive egocentricity . . . look for blunt affect* (emotionless expression on his face) when he discusses emotional issues, such as a relationship breakup or job loss.

As previously noted, psychopaths are not crazy; they know right from wrong, yet they act irrationally. With so much "controlled" violence surrounding sports and the shrewdness required for success in sports, Corporate America, and politics, we observe "industrial psychopaths," "jock psychopaths," and "political psychopaths" with little difficulty. The emotional damage to others caused by non-criminal psychopaths is striking. It seems **hubris** is a psychopathic virtue.

According to neurologist Dr. Martin Smedley of the UK, there is irrefutable biological basis (observed by brain scanning technology) showing *less emotional involvement* by "cool-coded" limbic system imagery, especially the amygdala, in the brains of psychopaths. Neuroscientists Dr. James Blair, Dr. Robert Hare, and others support the amygdala studies as well as anomalies identified in prefrontal lobes and temporal lobes.

Dr. Adrian Raine of UCLA believes within ten years *a computer chip* from microchip technology will offer a *bionic replacement for damaged prefrontal cortices* producing the worlds first "bionic brain".

◾ Brain-Body Chemistry—Chemical Precursors to Feeling

By themselves, drugs—any drugs—do not contain "highs," rather, they trigger "highs" already in place in the brain's "pleasure pathways", centers that evolved long ago to produce habituation to a wide array of pleasure, coincidentally, leading to propagation of the species. To a great extent, therefore, life depends on feeling pleasure.

In this section, we will analyze the neurochemistry for impact upon *rapacious behavior* observed in serial killers. We are persuaded by the FBI study on serial homicide that discovered the "one, indispensable ingredient"—the short fuse into rapacious behavior—is an *addiction to hardcore pornography* reflected in the FBI's *Criminal Personality Research Project* (1970), a research protocol of approximately 56 pages seeking answers behind serial homicide.

We believe evidence suggests for a second cause: *sexual repression* leading to obsessive curiosity caused by a hateful, domineering mother provides the perverse cognitive mapping responsible for twisting normal chemistry into the rapacious variety. Ted Bundy and a host of *organized* serial killers characterize the *addiction to pornography* variety, while Ed Gein and other organized and disorganized killers comprise the *sexual repression* category.

The following neurotransmitters are known to "jazz" behavior as *excitatory* neurochemistry and provide chemical underpinnings for a wide array of "jazzed" behavior including sexual obsession:

1. The Catecholamines: Norepinephrine (NE) and Dopamine (DA),
2. Phenylethylamine (PEA),
3. Androgenic hormone testosterone, and
4. Glutamate

Playing a vital role in synaptic cleft sequencing, **glutamate** is an *excitatory* neurotransmitter; yet research has confined the role glutamic to its functionality as observed in the action it performs in *ion conductance* and *intensifying neuronal firing rates*. Glutamate plays a major role in the brain's ability to strengthen synaptic connections, and appears to lie at the root of all learning, perhaps lying behind single cell memory. It accounts for the major neural damage of stroke as glutamate "fires" indiscriminately, causing extensive neural damage (unless blocked by an antagonist such as Naloxone®). Apparently, there is no "feeling" *per se* attached to glutamate, other than a person who feels "nervous" and lightheaded due to *MSG sensitivity* (monosodium glutamate), a derivative of glutamic acid.

Now we turn to the "feeling" chemistry that lies behind normal, abnormal, and rapacious behavior. Testosterone, a powerful hormone (often acting as a neurotransmitter in the brain as well as a hormone in the body) is our first stop.

■ The Chemical Id

The Androgenic Hormone—Testosterone

The anabolic steroid, *testosterone,* is the hormone of libido (sex drive) and aggression. Pure testosterone is perhaps the most powerful neurochemical in the body-brain. If an individual's *chromosomal sex* is the familiar male XY designation, the presence of testosterone acts to shape the developing embryo (soon to be known as a fetus) as a *"hard-wired" male brain.* In computer terms, the default setting under the influence of chromosomal sex XY is a male brain, morphology, and neurochemistry. To accomplish this differentiation, tiny embryonic ducts—**wolffian ducts**—develop under the influence of testosterone producing male internal structures and external genitalia, as well as "hard-wired" male brain circuitry.

It is well known in brain neuroscience that male and female brains are not the same in terms of localization and specificity of function.

Apparently, the defining difference in male/female brains is due to the presence or absence of testosterone. In the presence of testosterone, female ducts—**mullerian ducts**—existing alongside the Wolffian variety, are negated and absorbed into the body.

Social psychologists, criminologists, and behavioral scientists have long observed that elevated levels of testosterone have a positive correlation with *high crime rates*. Profilers and criminalists may not want to revisit a theory that continues to influence both science and science fiction, but the visit may be worthwhile. For example, in the early 20th century, Freud theorized **id** represented *sexual and aggressive tendencies* as well as *libido*—the sex drive.

Libido, Pleasure, and Sexual Addiction

Id (as libido) "operates" by virtue of the **pleasure principle**, or *mental fantasies* of eroticism or sexualized thinking. Today, we know testosterone is responsible for libido (sex drive) and the chemistry behind Freud's metaphorical id. Testosterone provides the powerful chemistry that lies behind sexual imagery, sexual fantasy, and of course, aggression. *Testosterone is the hormone of aggression.* Can a person become addicted to the feeling of libido caused by his own testosterone? This is precisely what occurs in sexual addiction.

The perfect organ of addiction is the human brain. It is both a manufacturer and depositor of powerful neurochemistry. In some individuals, habituation can lead very rapidly to addiction so that rational "choice" is replaced by feeling emotionally "compelled" to continue an activity, even though the addict knows the activity is illegal.

True sex addicts (not too far removed from normal teenagers!) are *addicted to the feeling* caused by surging testosterone and the chemistry that lies behind *feeling pleasure*—the feelings produced by fantasy, foreplay, and sex. The powerful neurotransmitter dopamine (DA), and to some extent other chemistry following in this section, account for the internal sense of the "thrilling high" of pleasure.

Before moving to a discussion of the powerful excitatory chemistry referred to as **catecholamines**—dopamine as a major source of feeling pleasure and **norepinephrine** (NE) as a "focuser" of jazzed activity—we conclude our discussion of testosterone with one final observation.

Driven by healthy levels of testosterone *in normally developed brains,* young males in their early twenties and mid-thirties are proactively building careers, staking their fortunes on hard work, dedication and focus, networking with colleagues and peers, planning new family members, or furthering their fortunes. It is normal that many males of this age category are college educated, and/or well on their way in graduate programs, law school, medical school, or developing skills and talents. They may have big dreams and follow those dreams aggressively.

Yet, it comes as no surprise that some otherwise happily married males may experience their first *extramarital affair* at this age, due, in part, to the ever-vigilant hormone with aphrodisiac qualities. While extra-martial sex may be morally questionable, it is not surprising and is certainly not considered a psychiatric disorder. (Psychology is not a moralistic discipline concerned about following the ethical or morally correct life. Instead, psychology is concerned with **existential** reality—ways we live authentic lives amid the stress and anxiety of modern problems.)

▪ Twenties to Thirties—A Potentially Dangerous Age Group

The quality of goals and expectations of normal 20 to mid-30 year old males stands in marked contrast to the depraved fantasies that plunge serial predators, who have *evidence of abnormal brain development and neurological damage,* into moral decadence. Normal males honor financial obligations and are careful to maintain contact with mentors, family, and friends. They are engaging in achievement-driven social behavior considered admirable for this age group. On the other hand, driven by the same levels of testosterone (crime statistics say "*elevated levels*"), the emerging sexual psychopath is engaging in dysfunctional, aberrant thinking. He's more likely to be a sullen loner (disorganized offender) who has squandered away formal schooling (he may be a high school dropout, more likely a college drop out). He has worked in a series of dead end jobs, probably lives with his parents, and is battling drug addiction. He may be a Peeping Tom and/or he may have had minor brushes with the law. Unquestionably, he is currently addicted to hardcore pornography and frequently visits sexually perverse sites online.

The "becoming" serial predator has never enjoyed a mutual, give and take relationship with a female peer. His alcoholic father may have introduced his son to prostitute, producing a confused and frustrated kid who only feels pleasure in his twisted fantasies. He anticipates crossing the line from fantasy into action. He spends hours in depraved fantasy. He seeks some measure of control in his life, but there is none. He desperately wants to show everybody how wrong they have been about him, how they have misjudged him, and how much he really has to offer. Yet, he depends on his parents or others for the necessities of life—food and shelter. When he should be thinking about his first serious job promotion or the birth of his first child, due to his ruined nervous system, he is ruminating about his first victim of rape and/or murder.

Testosterone, the hormone of sexual drive and aggression, is experienced internally on a vastly different plane than the one experienced by mainstream, normally adjusted young males. Neuroscientists know the "tracks" of neurochemistry "run" on the "rails" of thoughts set up by powerful *cognitive maps* of thinking, planning, imagination, and strategizing. The "maps" of thinking are set up by a history of parenting and social experiences, which profilers have found to be vacant, absent of nurturing and love. *Emotional scarcity* across a wide continuum characterizes the psychosocial, developmental history of serial killers.

▪ Sublimation of Libido

Due to dwindling hormonal levels of testosterone in men aged 40 or older, sexual and aggressive drives no longer predominate as the all-consuming torch it once did in ages 20s to mid-30s, the age group littered with serial predators. Around age fifty, normal males experience less sexually driven thoughts and are able to enjoy a wider circle of endeavors. **Sublimation** is the term invented by Freud to describe how a normal, aging male's thinking becomes more diffuse and varied instead of libidinal driven. In this way, he may achieve more socially admired creations in art, literature, or business acumen due to lower levels of the androgenic hormone. He might even write a textbook or two.

Theoretically, serial predators are incapable of experiencing sublimation due to neurological damage. Regardless, by age forty or fifty, most serial killers have been incarcerated for many years in prison, or they have been executed.

■ The Hormone Oxytocin (OXY)

As reported by Weatherford College criminal profiling student Rae Ellen Wooten, researcher Diane Witt, assistant professor of Psychology at Binghamton University (State University of New York), presented an article in the October 1998 edition of *Inside Binghamton University,* which provides an overview of the research linking oxytocin and socio-sexual behaviors. Witt contends . . ."The brain affects behavior, but behavior also affects the brain. The brain is very plastic (and) gonadal steroids provide a certain milieu in which other chemicals, like oxytocin, can affect the brain . . . in order to understand pathology, you first have to understand what the normal condition is . . . for instance . . . oxytocin plays a key role in bonding, even in species that are known to be antisocial."

Oxytocin (OXY), which is produced naturally in the hypothalamus, is a **neuropeptide**, which plays an important part in *maternal behavior and pair bonding,* and may be linked to socio-sexual influenced behaviors such as eating disorders, pedophilia, (and antisocial parenting)—child abuse and neglect. OXY receptors in the brain mediate numerous behavioral responses, including social, stress-related, learning and memory. OXY is a pro-social hormone that affects the brain as a result of interaction with the *gonadal steroids* such as estrogen, progesterone, testosterone and corticosterone. Studies show that *oxytocin* in females, as well as the closely related **vasopressin** in males, is the chemical behind *pair bonding.*

Research presents significant evidence that OXY can be classically conditioned to behavior, where touch (or inappropriate touch) is the CS— the conditioned stimulus that produces feeling. This is significant when bonding breaks down or is established inappropriately. According to Dr. Witt, "If there is a pathological condition—if too much oxytocin or a heightened sensitivity to oxytocin exists—there could be inappropriate pair bonding, such as pedophilia."

■ Dopamine: The Chemistry of Pleasure

Within the "pleasure pathways" of the medial forebrain bundle (*MFB*), a bundle of tightly packed interneurons (brain cells) of the **hypothalamus**, liberal receptors reside for the powerful neurotransmitter dopamine (DA). When DA is liberated in the brain (or in more abundance than inhibitor chemistry), *feelings of pleasure* predominate. This is exactly what serial predators experience during crimes—a heightened sense of pleasure and sexual energy—the "thrilling high" and perhaps sexual arousal to the point of a physical erection. Ted Bundy called it the "brutal urge" that drives rape and murder. One of two conditions can be theorized to occur. Either DA registers *low* in his brain, which produces an intense desire to feel any pleasure he can *by extreme measures* such as rape or murder, or observed as *overkill*. Another possible answer is DA liberates quickly at binding sites producing the "thrilling high" that only comes from *extreme behavior*—raping and killing. In either condition, *dopaminergic* sites are activated producing sexualized pleasure.

Dr. Olds and Dopamine

A *physiological psychologist* (precursor to neuropsychologists), Dr. James Olds, discovered the powerful effects of MFB and dopamine by accident in the last 1960s. He received permission to implant electrodes directly into the brain of a dangerous mental patient who was both homicidal and suicidal. One of the micro-thin electrodes traversed the center of the MFB. The patient could stimulate three areas of his brain by pushing one of three buttons on his belt connected to the electrodes. He favored the middle button (the one connecting to his MFB) so much that he had to be disconnected from the electrodes due to over-stimulation. The patient spent hours stimulating his own MFB and received the equivalent of one organism after another! Why would he want to stop? From that surreptitious discovery, Dr. Olds appropriately labeled the MFB of the hypothalamus the "pleasure pathway."

Erotic & Pornographic

We must remember that dopamine lies behind all pleasure—whether it's due to normal sexuality (whatever that is!), or *rapacious sexuality* from the mind of serial predators. Apparently, the difference revolves around the *perception* of what is sexually "pleasuring". Is it consensual and nurturing to the initiator, to the receiver? Apparently, "degrading, domineering, and rapacious" describe sexuality that is stimulating to serial predators due to their neurologically damaged brain and perverted cognitive mapping. Since *cognitive focus* determines parameters of perception and interest, focus defines what is stimulating and what is not. Could forcible rape and sadistic murder somehow be eroticized in the mind of killers? Strong anecdotal evidence exists that the vehicle for eroticized bondage, pain, and degradation comes from viewing similar behavior in pornographic films, the *one common addiction of serial predators*.

◨ Speculative Logic—The Influence of Pornography Upon Rapacious Behavior

Pornography (literally "writing about prostitutes") is defined as the depiction of erotic behavior (esp. pictures, films, or movies) intended to cause sexual excitement. **Hardcore porn** focuses on sadistic rape fantasies, sexualized violence, manipulation, bondage, and degradation. To experienced investigators, many serial crimes seem to have been committed by perpetrators who just finished watching hardcore porn.

Snuff movies (the word first appearing in dictionaries in 1975) refer to sensationalistic films depicting violence and real (rather than staged) murder of a participant. Recently, a movie *8 millimeter,* starring Nicolas Cage, addressed this theme.

We address three questions regarding the purported role of pornography in serial crimes. What are the expectations of viewers who watch pornographic movies, specifically those with neurologically damaged brains? How are women depicted in such movies? What kind of relationship exists between the participants of hardcore porn movies?

Regarding the expectations of viewing hardcore porn (XX-rated or XXX-rated), viewers expect *explicit sex acts* with a variety of partners in a variety of positions with oral, anal, and/or vaginal sex. Group sex, lesbian sex, and orgies might also be anticipated. Viewers expect to be sexually stimulated; most viewers masturbate numerous times as they view naked bodies engaging in explicit sex. Sexually obsessed or sadistic males might force their girlfriends to watch and perform as a female porn "actress". Some females may comply to avoid being beaten or raped. It's possible that some females enjoy the sexualized themes, but most often, even compliant co-offenders, find them degrading and "sick."

In hardcore porn, (as well as soft-core porn) the real danger to occasional viewers is the manner in which females are exploited. Females are almost always portrayed as willing participants in even the most exotic sexual acts imaginable. They are portrayed as around-the-clock, sexually receptive *nymphs* (derived from the term **nymphomania** denoting females with excessive sexual desire, a psychiatric condition). Or, they are portrayed as harboring rape fantasies themselves, or being willing to be dominated by a "real" man, a man unafraid of "taking what he wants".

Relationships between participants in hardcore porn are domination by the female. Yet, males get what they want from compliant female "sexual slaves" or, a female sexual dominatrix "services" any number of compliant males. The message is a dangerous one: females are to be dominated, exploited, and controlled. Sexual experimentation is encouraged. Female porn stars are paid high salaries; males receive a paltry salary. Porn films focus on the female. Porn films depict females to exist for the total pleasure of males.

◨ The Rapacious Twist

The rapacious "twist" on normal brain chemistry may occur in the following scenario: a male with a neurologically damaged brain overly influenced by reptilian brain centers (with a history of violent antisocial parenting) feels angry and rejected from his emotionally vacant childhood. Driven by revenge and anger for his dysfunctional life, his fantasies become sexualized by an addiction to pornography, or in the alternative, hyper-sexualized by *sexual repression* from a domineering mother. It is our contention that his addiction to porn, sexual repression, and other chemical addictions (cocaine, "crank," or alcohol) acts, through perverted cognitive mapping, to transform neurochemistry into the rapacious variety.

In conclusion, it appears the "script" for many serial rapes and murders are inspired and motivated by rapists and killers deeply addicted to pornography. Serial killer Ted Bundy blamed his murderous fantasies directly on pornography. According to Bundy

> "I am not a social scientist. I haven't run any surveys, but I've been in prison a long time. I've met many men motivated to commit murders just like me, and every one of them had an addiction to pornography. It's true. The FBI's own study on serial homicide agrees, pornography is the one single thread that runs through serial homicide."

We now turn to the chemical that lies behind initiating mental focus, interest, and perception, the catecholamine norepinephrine (NE)—the cognitive "focuser."

■ NE: Focuser of "Jazzed" Behavior

Norepinephrine (NE) (and to some extent DA since it is "made" from NE) lies behind focus, attention, interest, commitment, and resolve. Together, DA/NE lies behind feeling jazzed, inspired, and provides the energy behind motivation and resolve. As we have seen, DA/NE lies behind addiction. Taking "speed" liberates NE (jazzed feeling) and DA (pleasurable feelings), hence we feel "jazzed pleasure" from *stimulants;* cocaine liberates DA as a *euphorostimulant,* hence we feel "euphoric" and "stimulated". There is no reason to doubt DA/NE's role in the addiction of serial predators.

Normal behavior (as well as a normal personality) occurs because DA/NE is balanced by other brain chemistry, notably serotonin (5-HT) and GABA. For example, when DA is abnormally high, or not sufficiently mitigated by inhibitory chemistry, **schizophrenia**, a psychotic disorder characterized by a severe thought and behavioral disorder may result. "Crank" addicts, individuals addicted to *methamphetamine,* or "speed" liberate large amounts of DA/NE in the process of addiction, resulting in almost voiding out reserves of DA/NE; often, they display symptoms of paranoid schizophrenia. Perhaps, it is not too farfetched to suggest that "crank" addiction matches the fierce addiction to serial crime, since only 6% of "crank" addicts recover (compared to 0% of serial predators). The recovery rate of cocaine addiction is higher. Diagnosed as paranoid schizophrenics, the rapacious crimes of serial killers David Berkowitz and Richard Chase were psychotic, a departure for most serial killers who know exactly what they're doing.

Similarly, with NE dominance, behavior can become excessively *hypervigilant,* as observed in *obsessive-compulsive* behavior seen in repetitive crimes such as stalking victims and serial offenses. It can be postulated that during *mens rea,* NE cascades in the CNS as the "torch" of motivation, while **adrenaline** reinforces imminent action in the body. Hence with DA and NE in dominance, we are alert, attentive, focused, and driven whether we are students eager to learn, or teachers "jazzed" to teaching, or serial rapists and killers displaying rapacious behavior.

The area of the midbrain known as the *substantia nigra* manufactures DA for delivery to the *caudate nucleus* of the basal ganglia—four deeply placed masses of gray matter within each cerebral hemisphere, including the *amygdala*. It is in this region where fine movements and muscle tone are controlled. Evidence for dopaminergic failure in this region can be observed in the movement disorder known as **Parkinson's Disease.** Dopaminergic neurons extend from the ventral tegmentum in the midbrain to the part of the limbic system concerned with *emotionality and reward,* the hypothalamus.

■ Blocking Reuptake—Liberating Brain Chemistry

CNS *euphorostimulants* such as cocaine, methamphetamines (speed), and methylphenidate (Ritalin), liberate DA by a chemical process known as blocking reuptake. **Blocking reuptake** is a neural mechanism well known to psychopharmacology. It operates by interfering with presynaptic vesicles attempting to "reclaim" leftover neurotransmitter chemistry in the synapse. The process prevents or blocks vesicles as molecular "pumps" from reclaiming contents of the synapse after receptor binding. Unrecalled, the synaptic chemistry is used immediately to augment and stabilize receptor chemistry that preceded it in receptor sites.

Therefore, "blocking reuptake" translates into liberating chemistry for immediate use in the synaptic cleft, so that a sustained release is possible. Such a condition occurs when cocaine liberates dopamine; hence, cocaine "blocks reuptake" of DA and provides efficacy of addiction. The cocaine addict is addicted to the "thrilling high" from his own dopamine. (Conversely, simple *blocking* neurochemistry means chemistry is "blocked" and made unavailable at the synapse. This "mitigating" action is due to blocking receptors post-synaptically. An example of "blocking" is observed in the treatment of schizophrenia with the antipsychotic drug, *Thorazine,* which prevents DA from binding, hence blocking DA or lessening dopaminergic activity.)

It is not too far-fetched to purpose that serial predators are addicted to their own DA/NE much like the cocaine addict or speed "freak." Pornographic films no longer "work" like doing the real thing.

■ Serotonin (5-HT)—The Four Cs

Cool, Calm, Collected, and Confident

Serotonin (5-HT) influences behavior that is calm, cool, collected, and confident. Leaders, popular individuals we universally trust, and individuals with pleasing personalities who "disarm" others by setting them at ease are due to 5-HT dominance. Former President Bill Clinton possessed gifts of 5-HT liberation. Regardless of his *hubristic* troubles, the homeland economy flourished under his confidence-inspiring guidance. When he gave his televised messages, we believed him, even when he said "I never had sex with that intern."

When the major *inhibitory neurotransmitter* in the CNS, **GABA**, is at normal or elevated levels, it produces *anti-anxiety effects* and calming behavior. In this way, GABA/5-HT provides *stabilizing behavior* in overall personality functioning. While DA/NE is excitatory and produces "jazzed" behavior, 5-HT/GABA is inhibitory and produces "calming" behavior. This produces the well-known "seesaw of mind"—the better the balance between inhibitory versus excitatory chemistry—the more likely an individual is free from depression, mania, eating disorders, and personality disorders.

5-HT is an inhibitor of activity and behavior. It increases sleep time and reduces aggression and sexual activity. Most of the brain's *serotonergic* cells are located in the *raphe,* or the seam-like union of the two halves of the brain stem, of the reptilian brain. 5-HT is an ancient neurotransmitter found in all primates.

Recent evidence of *low brain serotonin (5-HT) and elevated levels of testosterone* may be the neural "cocktail" of biochemistry behind psychopathy. Finally, irreversible, neurological damage to critical areas of the brain, especially the prefrontal cortex, amygdala, and cerebellum categorize the deformed brains of sexual predators. Clearly, sexual psychopaths (or "Rambo" killers), detailed in Chapter Seven do not have normal brains.

Personality & Low 5-HT Levels

Low 5-HT levels have been linked to the following:

1. Disturbances of mood,
2. Increased appetite,
3. Premenstrual Syndrome (or PMS),
4. Depression and suicide, and
5. Cravings associated with eating disorders and alcoholism.

Studies in North America at UCLA and in the UK link elevated 5-HT levels in males to a feeling of *power and dominance,* based on primate studies. Also, 5-HT imbalance can occur in males who consume too much alcohol. They want to fight anyone and everyone. Since low levels of 5-HT are associated with low self-esteem and feeling "empty" inside, perhaps, 5-HT/GABA is low in the spinal fluid of serial offenders. They may appear in persona to be calm, cool, collected, and confident but we know they feel wretched, empty, and consumed with rage on the inside.

Psychotropic medications such as Prozac, Zoloft, and Deseryl are examples of **SSRIs** (**selective serotonin reuptake inhibitors**), which allow a sustained release of the soothing neurotransmitter 5-HT into post-synaptic receptors. In the language we have learned, SSRIs *block reuptake* of serotonin, liberating it for post-synaptic use. In contrast, toxic agents that destroy serotonergic cells have been observed in so-called "designer drugs" like ecstasy, (MDMA), which erode brain tissue in the reptilian brain.

◼ The Amino Acid Neurotransmitters

Neurotransmitters in the majority of *ion-channeled linked receptors* (fast-acting synapses), are also the molecular building blocks of proteins known as *amino acids*. By name they are aspartate, glycine, glutamate, and gamma-aminobutyric acid or GABA. Having already provided a discussion on glutamate, we now turn to GABA.

◼ Gamma-Aminobutyric Acid (GABA)

Similar to 5-HT, the amino acid GABA is an *inhibitor of brain activity*. Arousal, aggression, and anxiety are reduced along with other hyper-vigilant behaviors. GABA is found primarily in the hippocampus and amygdala as well as the hypothalamus. GABA is the major *inhibitory neurotransmitter* in the CNS. We rest, sleep, rejuvenate, and experience less anxiety due to balanced GABA.

Low-level GABA has been associated with the following, anxiety, insomnia, epilepsy, and Huntington's Disease (inherited movement and cognitive-loss disorder). At the tissue and cellular level, **anxiety** can be conceptualized as excessive firing in specific brain areas, especially the limbic system. When GABA is disseminated in the cleft, it leads to its own depletion, the "messenger is slain," so to speak.

To reverse the depletion, the presence of a prescribed drug such as diazepam (Valium®), or other benzodiazepines enhances GABA binding by liberating GABA through blocking reuptake. This activity intensifies *anti-anxiety* effects. Therefore, when GABA registers low in the CNS, anxiety is experienced.

In the treatment of stress and/or anxiety, *benzodiazepines* are the drugs of choice for liberating GABA at the synaptic level. Valium®, Librium®, Xanax®, Ativan®, and Buspar® promote GABAergic transmission.

Rapacious behavior presents itself as a depletion of 5-HT/GABA at post-synaptic sites. In such a condition, the person's behavior would be characterized as anxious, unsettled, and perhaps "nerve-racked."

◼ Endogenous Opioid Peptides (Endorphins)

Endogenous opioid peptides (*endorphins*) are naturally-occurring internal opioids, related pharmacologically to morphine, with a contraction meaning, "morphine within." Natural CNS receptor sites allow for powerful opioid drugs to bind naturally in the brain. Endorphins are released in response to the following:

1. pain,
2. vigorous exercise, and
3. sexual behavior

Internal opioids acting as neurotransmitters and *external* narcotic drugs act similarly as both have an affinity for opioid receptors. Drugs that mimic natural brain opioids and share an affinity for their receptors are known as an **agonist**. They are derivatives of opium such as morphine, heroin, codeine, and Percodan®. Synthetic compounds that resemble morphine such as Demerol® and Darvon® act on binding sites as though they were natural opioid chemistry. The rewarding effects of opioids are mediated by the *dopaminergic system*—the system of feeling pleasure. It is not farfetched or unreasonable to assume craving the endorphin "rush" in the nervous systems of serial offenders who derive pleasure from inflicting pain (often vigorously administered) through sexualized acts.

We presume 5-HT/GABA to register low in the spinal fluid of a serial killer due to neurological damage of his brain brought about by attachment anxiety, poor parenting, and developmental assaults where he feels unloved and unwanted. Perhaps, the *fait accompli* of sexualized, rapacious behavior and the "thrilling high" derived from acts of rape and murder are due to the intoxicating and ambivalent "rush" of feelings associated with:

1. **Analgesic** effects of anticipated endorphin "rush," and
2. *Erotic pleasure* derived from peaking DA and testosterone,
3. Specificity of phenylethylamine (PEA) "rush" to his chosen victim, and
4. Serotonin (5-HT) depletion, producing anxiety and ultimately the "empty" feeling of non-fulfillment.

▪ PEA (Phenylethylamine)—Chemistry Behind Attraction

A biogenic amine (a compound), **PEA (phenylethylamine)** (fugh-neth-lugh-meen) functions as a neurotransmitter. PEA resembles amphetamine in pharmacological properties. Some researchers suggest that it may account for the so-called *romantic rush* associated with the initial attraction experienced between individuals. PEA may account for the behavior and feelings associated with welcomed *flirtatious behavior* and the anticipation of intimacy or sex. It lies behind childish playfulness and the desire to be close to and touch others in flirtatious ways. Similar to the natural rush of PEA, analogous feelings can be obtained externally by the use of amphetamines, which produce the effects of "aroused pleasure." This occurs by liberating DA/NE receptors.

A serial predator trolling for more victims experiences heightened sexualized perception when he finds a victim that fits his prototype. Just like a normal brain chemistry conditioned to eroticism, brain chemistry conditioned to the pornographic "mindset" experiences erotic, rapacious thoughts toward individuals intended as victims. Apparently, PEA jazzes the serial killer's brain when he fantasizes about or actually sees his targeted victim, just like a lizard or snake hiding in the grass watching the movements of his next meal nearby. It is similar to how a grizzly stands practically motionless for hours, waiting for the precise moment to attack his targeted victim, so the organized sexual predator patiently drives around strategically searching for his next victim.

◼ Oxytocin (OXY) & Vasopressin

The *posterior pituitary gland* secretes two important regulating hormones. For males, vasopressin appears to lie behind social bonding, while oxytocin (OXY), known as the "cuddle chemical," accomplishes the same in females. Studies with primates show convincing results. When OXY is blocked by chemistry, primate moms do not bond with their offspring; in some instances they try to harm them.

Could an underdeveloped, immature brain caused by incompetent and hateful parenting cause a glitch in vasopressin? Why not? The serial predator has a lot going against him; perhaps the most devastating is *retarded* brain development (neurologically damaged brain) caused by incompetent and hateful parenting, developmental glitches, and addiction; hence the normal functioning of vasopressin is mitigated—serial rapists and killers do not bond with other human beings.

◼ Acetylcholine (Ach)

The ubiquitous neurotransmitter and parasympathetic nervous system agent, **Ach (acetylcholine)** (ugh-seat-ugh-co-leen), is responsible for some distinctive human characteristics such as:

1. conservation of energy,
2. attention and memory,
3. thirst,
4. sexual behavior,
5. mood, and
6. REM sleep.

Much of the brain's Ach is produced in the basal forebrain. Since Ach has been implicated in memory and learning, cholinergic neurons are found in the hippocampus and cortex, where tissue areas for learning, memory formation and retrieval exist.

The rapacious "twist" on cholinergic chemistry could have a depleting action upon mood unless enhanced by the excitement of encountering a new victim.

■ Soluble-Gas Neurotransmitters

Nitric oxide and *carbon monoxide* have recently been discovered as a class of small-molecule neurotransmitters. However, they do not act like other neurotransmitters. They are produced in the neural cytoplasm and immediately diffuse through the cell membrane into the extracellular fluid and then easily pass into nearby cells. They do so because they are soluble in lipids (fats). They pose a special challenge because they are so difficult to study. They stimulate the production of *second messenger neurotransmitters* and are immediately broken down, lasting only a few seconds.

■ Second Messengers

G-Protein linked receptors are more prevalent than ion-channel linked receptors. *Ion-channel linked receptors* are linked to chemically activated ion channels so when linkage occurs the ion channel usually opens or closes quickly. The result is to induce immediate postsynaptic potential so that *biochemical action occurs quickly.*

In some cases when a neurotransmitter binds to a G-protein linked receptor, a subunit of the adjacent G-protein breaks away. One result may be to trigger the synthesis of a second messenger chemical. Neurotransmitters such as DA/NE and 5-HT/GABA are considered first messengers so that behavior relating to *long-term effects exists due to* second messengers.

G-protein linked receptors in contrast to ion-channeled receptors produce *slower, more sustained, more diffuse, and more varied effects, hence longer lasting feeling and emotion.*

Second messenger transmission is the cerebral "tracks" that sustained mood "runs" upon. In such instances, a person can be happy and well adjusted for months and years at a time. In contrast, the same is true for depression, dysthymia, or a psychopathic personality. With ion-channeled transmission only, the "peeks and valleys" of emotion would occur, practically minute by minute. Careful consideration must be given to the powerful chemistry underlying positive thinking, short-term goals, and laughter.

Imagine the mindset of a serial predator with a steady diet of pornography, triggering rape and/or murderous fantasies, who is *"locked" into repetitive and ritualistic behavior largely due to second messenger programming.*

Imagine the mind of serial killer Arthur Shawcross.

PREDATOR PROFILE (5-2)

Arthur Shawcross
"The Rochester Night Stalker"

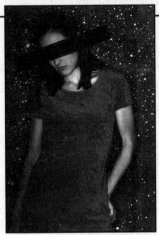

Alternative Monikers:

"The Rochester Strangler"
"The Geneese Killer"

Time Span:

1972 to1989. 1990 captured

Physical Description:

Bald, overweight, middle-aged white male.

Offenses Prior to Killing:

Often beat up children in the neighborhood
Set a paper mill on fire
Stole from local businesses
Broke into houses
While in Vietnam, he raped and killed Vietnamese women and children

Victimology:

His victims were mainly white females (eleven in all) who were prostitutes or homeless. He picked them up in a car borrowed from a woman he was having a sexual affair with. He drove them to a secluded spot by a river. He had sex with them, strangled them, and returned later to satisfy his desire for necrophilia. He often cannibalized the dead body. He had a fetish for oral sex.

Current Status:

Shawcross is now serving a sentence in prison of 450 years. While in prison he was caught selling autographs and paintings.

General Background:

Arthur Shawcross had a horrible life growing up. As a child his mother did hateful things to him like sodomize him with a broomstick. He was also told to have oral sex with his aunt who taught him how to do it. This is where his fetish for oral sex came from. As a child he was caught having sex with his sister whom she denies to this day that it happened. He was caught once by his girlfriend's brother performing oral sex on her. The only way he would not tell on them was if Shawcross performed oral sex on him, too. That was his first homosexual encounter. Until age eight he was a chronic bed wetter.

Shawcross was a very good student in grade school and had an easy time making good grades. The only thing holding him back was the fact that he did not like the other kids that he was there with and he would often pick on them until he made them cry. Shawcross never really had any friends and he was thought to be a loner.

While growing up he became more and more violent and this is when he began to break into houses and buildings. He still wet the bed and became more withdrawn from the world. During this time at the age of fourteen he began to have oral sex with his cousin and sister. Shawcross still had his virginity to speak of which might have suggested that he could not keep an erection.

In 1968 he joined the army and was shipped off to Vietnam. While in Vietnam he became more violent. When he stumbled upon Vietnamese women and children, he often tortured them. He tied them up and raped them repeatedly. After he was finished, he decapitated the corpses, leaving them for the Viet Cong to find.

After he left Vietnam he came home and married a woman he had recently met. He was employed at a cheese factory, which he set on fire amounting to his second arson. Shawcross was later arrested and sentenced on two counts of arson. While in prison he was raped by two African Americans whom he later retaliated against. He was sent to another prison where he saved a guard's life and was granted parole.

After returning to life after prison he took up fishing as a hobby. He found a fishing buddy who turned out to be a victim. The two were seen together several times. When the boy went missing, authorities found his body and went looking for Shawcross. He later admitted to eating the boy's genitals and heart. Another child went missing within a month or two. With this case the police had enough evidence to arrest and convict Arthur Shawcross.

Shawcross stayed in jail until he was finally "deemed fit to return to society". He went back to the town where he had murdered the two children. The citizens ran him out of town as a known sex offender. He moved on and married again. A year later, Shawcross started murdering prostitutes and homeless women. He was apprehended in 1990 and convicted of eleven murders. He was sentenced to four hundred and fifty years in prison.

Student Contributors:

Chasidy Wilson, Meagon Hurst, and Sandra Forrester

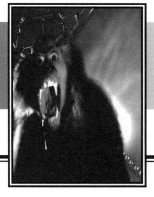

Aftermath

I. Word Scholar

Define the following words from *The Word Scholar Glossary.*

  1. Brain stem _____

  2. Prefrontal lobes _____

  3. Limbic system _____

  4. Association cortices _____

  5. Dopamine (DA) _____

  6. Norepinephrine (NE) _____

  7. Oxytocin (OXY) _____

  8. Nymphomania _____

  9. Serotonin (5-HT) _____

  10. GABA _____

II. The Forensic Lab

Compose a one page paper addressing: What do you perceive to be the specific neurochemicals in creating rapacious mind? What causes otherwise normal chemistry to become rapacious?

CHAPTER 6

Netherworld: Antisocial Parenting & Adolescent Psychopathy

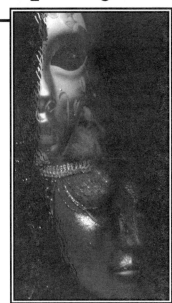

" *The head inside the jar had been severed neatly close beneath the jaw. It faced her . . . the mouth was open and the tongue protruded slightly, very gray . . . Now, at this moment, sitting in this old car with a head and some mice, she could think clearly, and she was proud of that.* **"**

—*Silence of the Lambs*
Thomas Harris

> "And not infrequently parents who are professional people—doctors, lawyers, club women, and philanthropists—who lead lives of strict orderliness and decorum but yet lack love, send children into the world who are as undisciplined and destructive and disorganized as any child from an impoverished and chaotic home."
>
> **—M. Scott Peck, M.D. (The Road Less Traveled)**

This book is ultimately about *causes* told through the *effects* of sexual psychopathy. It's about parenting, or rather, the effects of *toxic parenting* in the development of children. Interviews with incarcerated sexual psychopaths provide background information regarding horrific family milieus—the breeding ground for sexual predators. *Along with all violent criminals, parents of sexual psychopaths are the true criminals of society.* They create Netherworld and the children from it who are destroyers.

The faceless, pathetic parents of criminals litter the background in anonymity. Yet, they are responsible to a great extent for raising antisocial misfits. Severely dysfunctional themselves, they seem confused when asked how their son or daughter turned out "so bad." Herein lies a glaring flaw in the perception of antisocial parents. As emotionally damaged individuals, they perpetuate deviance by "setting up" pathology in family milieus, ensuring that another generation of dysfunction continues. Rapacious parents—parents who prey upon their young in hateful and abusive ways—are too drug-addled, too emotionally dysfunctional, or emotionally absent to care for themselves, much less a child, who demands clearheadedness and good-heartedness to have a fighting chance at normalcy.

■ Netherworld: Toxic Parenting

Surviving horrific parental abuses themselves, **toxic parenting** is continued by constructing elaborate defenses against self-hatred, anxiety, and anger. Emotional defenses such *denial, rationalization,* and *regression* temporarily defuses anxiety caused by knowing "deep down" the child is not loved and not wanted. The child interferes with parents' addictions and perversities.

According to Freud, the master architect of emotional defenses, *denial* operates like conscious *repression.* Parents deny that they are the cause of their children's problems, just like the alcoholic who denies his excessive drinking is a problem, even though he loses everything and hits rock bottom. Dysfunctional parents reason: Why should we change if we're not the problem? Obviously, looking into the mirror and seeing themselves as dysfunctional parents is just too emotionally painful. So they use denial or "construct" more elaborate defenses. The defense of *rationalization* employs a flimsy excuse for every problem. *Nothing is ever the fault of incompetent and antisocial parents.* The problem is always "other people" and "the kid."

Children grow up in the image of their parents. From incompetent parenting—uninvolved, passive, unimaginative, addicted—the minimally-skilled parents whose kids "get their way"—come garden variety psychopaths and other social misfits. *From toxic (antisocial) parents come sexual psychopaths, the serial killers and rapists of society.*

The defense of *regression* allows psychopaths—both parents and the "becoming" psychopathic child—to remain dependent, immature, and pathetic slaves to emotional dysfunction.

In our nomenclature, *incompetent parents* are parents who do not, in general, rear criminals but, nonetheless, deeply scar their children emotionally thorough inadequate emotional expressions of love, caring, and nurturing. They display minimal parental skills. They often berate their children with verbal abuse and threats. Garden-variety psychopaths—the severe male narcissists and female histrionics and borderlines—come from incompetent parents who display ambivalence in discipline, emotional involvement, and love. Children from these homes often grow up with *addiction problems* related to chemical abuse, attempting self-medication. Incompetent parents also "smother" their children with *faux*-love or completely spoil them rotten.

When troubled teenagers (who often become sexually promiscuous) have their own children, they perpetuate incompetent parenting by repeating the lessons from their own dysfunctional parenting. Why shouldn't this be the case? Usually, they have not devoted time to learning effective parenting skills from college courses or from local mental health organizations. Why should they? Like all psychopaths with narcissistic or histrionic features, *they have all the answers*. In reality, they have all the wrong answers.

■ Emotional Nihilism

In our nomenclature, *antisocial parents* rear violent criminals and sexual psychopaths. They go beyond leaving emotional scars inflicted by incompetent parents by producing *irreversible neurological damage* in their children's central nervous system from severe physical and sexual abuse, hateful emotional treatment, and/or neglect.

Emotional **nihilism** characterizes the perception of sexual psychopaths (and their parents) who view people and morality as "nothing" worthy of disposal. Without love and nurturing throughout their lives, it is no wonder that *they feel destruction is desirable since existence is meaningless.*

The current chapter is an antisocial parental "script" for the development of sons with sexual psychopathy, and for daughters who become prostitutes, criminal offenders, and killers. On the flip side, it's about what to avoid when parents seek to raise emotionally normal children. Following the "recipe" of deviant parental "scripts," sweet and innocent children with all of the promise of excelling in life and finding happiness in normal pursuits is transformed into a disgusting, antisocial misfit. Hateful, antisocial parenting results in molding a cold-blooded "reptile" hiding behind a human face.

As a full-blown serial killer, authorities look back after his capture to a history of oppositional deviant behavior and most likely, the homicidal triad of *enuresis, cruelty,* and *pyromania*. Red flags of psychopathy litter his home and school milieus. Due to brain differences related to gender, and other unknown reasons, daughters raised by antisocial parenting usually turn anger and humiliation inward, rather than outward. (Female serial killers, along with adolescent "Rambo" killers who kill kids and adults, will be featured in the following chapter, Psychology of Perversion, Chapter Seven).

■ Childhoods of Violence

In the late 1970s, the FBI's 57-page *Criminal Personality Research Profile* asked 36 incarcerated serial killers to talk about childhood influences. For the first time, investigators were allowed insight into the horrific milieus of violent childhoods. What they discovered is not surprising. Serial killers are *conditioned to become violent criminals in severely dysfunctional homes by antisocial (toxic) parenting*. In this regard, sins of *omission* (what parents failed to do) are just as glaring as sins of *commission* (what parents did). According to the experts, sexual psychopaths, as well as garden variety psychopathic personality, are reared, not born. Neuroscientists do not expect to find a gene of psychopathy.

The following criminal characteristics have been extracted from the aforementioned questionnaire from violent and traumatic childhoods marked by antisocial parenting. Twenty-three salient factors are presented in no special order.

Twenty-three Characteristics of Antisocial (Toxic) Parenting

1. In the survey, half of the incarcerated offenders (18 men) had *mental illness* in their immediate family.
2. Half of the subjects had parents who were involved in *some form of criminality.*
3. Nearly 70% (25 men) had a family *history of alcohol or drug abuse.*
4. All serial killers—all 36—had a history of *serious emotional abuse.*
5. All the killers had developed into *sexually dysfunctional adults,* unable to sustain "a mature, consensual relationship" with another adult.
6. From birth to age seven (an important time for *maternal bonding*), relationships between the killers and their mothers were "uniformly cool, distant, unloving, and neglectful".
7. All 36 killers experienced *mental and/or physical abuse.*
8. From a young age, all 36 offenders' behavior was ignored, and few if any, limits were imposed on behavior, leading to an *egocentric* view of the world.
9. Over 40% (14 men) were physically beaten.
10. Over 70% (25 men) reported, "witnessing or participating in *sexually stressful events* when young" (sexual abuse, fondling, attempted rape, or rape).
11. In all 36 offenders, *no sense of familial attachments*—not feeling an emotional belonging to family—resulted in feeling "lonely and isolated."
12. In all 36 offenders, from ages eight-twelve years of age, "negative and destructive influences of earlier stages were exacerbated". No strong, influential adult "rescued" any of them.
13. Half of the offenders (18 men) had *absent fathers*—some died, others became incarcerated. Some fathers left through divorce or abandonment during adolescent years.
14. More than 75% (27 men) reported *autoerotic fantasies* as preadolescents. Half (18 men) reported *rape fantasies* occurring between the ages of 12–14.
15. In all cases, the sexualized nature of crimes showed *every single subject was sexually dysfunctional*.
16. As a rule, the offenders, as young adolescents, experienced a confusing mix of "compulsive masturbation, bed-wetting, and nightmares."
17. Although some of the killers had high IQs, none performed well in school; most hated school.
18. In all 36 cases, energy was directed to "negative outlets" that consumed them such as drugs, vandalism, burglary, and pornography, since no positive stimulation came from home or school.

19. In all 36 cases, perverse, sexualized fantasies fuelled the killers' murderous acts—hence, all serial murders have underlying, unresolved sexual themes.
20. In all cases, due to extensive sexual fantasies, *victims are depersonalized* as objects—the person is "evicted from his body" as one killer phrased it.
21. Sexual urges are *disconnected* from affection and tender emotion.
22. Sexualized, deviant *cognitive maps* stimulate perversity that pornography only temporarily satisfies, "forcing" offenders to actually confront live victims.
23. Pre-crime "triggers" or stressors exists—some perceived loss, a job, money problems, or a vociferous argument—that escalated rapidly into violence. Afterward, most offenders are both frightened and thrilled, but mostly thrilled.

SOURCE: *Whoever Fights Monsters* (Ressler, 1992).

◾ Milieus Characterized by "Predator Parenting"

1. Richard Trenton Chase "The Vampire Killer"

Parenting milieu characterized by anger, mental illness, drug addiction, physical abuse, and alcoholism.

Chase grew up in a household of anger, mental illness, and alcoholism. His mother was an alcoholic and a drug addict who displayed signs of schizophrenia. His father was a strict disciplinarian who used physical abuse as punishment and as a way to "solve problems." At an early age, Chase was a fire-starter.

As he grew older his crimes escalated to more serious offences; he showed no remorse for his misconduct. As an adolescent, he was a loner showing signs of psychopathy—displaying deviant fantasies. He was never perceived as a "ladies man" and was ridiculed for being sexually impotent. Often, he found dead animals and brought them home. He likely cannibalized them. Once, he injected rabbit blood into his own veins. The procedure made him deathly ill. Somehow, he survived. Eventually, doctors diagnosed Chase as a paranoid schizophrenic, suffering from somatic (bodily) delusions—he felt his blood would turn to powder without blood transfusions (comprising his blood fetish).

Chase is one of the few sexual killers who actually had a psychiatric diagnosis. Most serial killers are not psychotic; they know exactly what they're doing.

Dahmers father shows
no emotion.
No bonding w/ father.

2. Jeffrey Lionel Dahmer
"The Milwaukee Cannibal"

*Parenting milieu characterized by physical and emotional aban-
donment issues from emotionally distant parents, possible molestation from a neighbor, homosexual fantasies, road-kill autopsies,
and alcoholism.*

Born 10 years after Chase in 1960, Jeffrey Lionel Dahmer grew up
with unhappily married parents. They spent most of their waking hours
in verbal sparring. The family moved often during the early years of
his life.

From birth, Dahmer had medical problems. He was born with broken legs and had to wear splints until he was three years old. He couldn't
walk until he was two. Then, he had to have help standing up. At the age
of four, he received surgery for a hernia. Causing considerable pain,
Dahmer recalled the experience as "embarrassing." Erroneously, he
thought the doctor had amputated his penis; years later, he felt this experience emotionally scarred him. As he grew up he was quiet and kept to
himself. At the age of eight, it was rumored that a neighbor boy molested
him, although nothing was proven. However, it was at this age Dahmer
became introverted and behaviorally disruptive.

In school, he made a spectacle of himself in class as the class clown.
Often, he ran down the hallways of his school shouting and waving his
arms—peers referred to his behavior as "doing a Dahmer." Teachers considered him to be a bright child, but he only managed average grades. He
never liked school.

As an adolescent, Dahmer began experimenting with the dead carcasses of animals. This macabre event coincided with the start of puberty.
He brought home road kill and performed autopsies on them. Since his
father was a chemist, Dahmer used his knowledge of acids to wear the tissue from bones. At this point, he began to fantasize what humans would
look like on the inside.

Dahmer was discovering that along with his puberty he was becoming attracted to men, and only men. He didn't know how to handle his
urges—he dared not mention this to his parents—so he began to drink in
an effort to self-medicate. He was plagued by the fantasy of lying next to
an unconscious person, someone who could meet his needs, but not telling
anyone or asking anything in return. He became a fierce alcoholic, trying
to suppress his thoughts, but eventually, he was compelled to act out and
murder his first victim. Dahmer hid in the woods one day soon after he
could no longer control his urges. He hoped to disable a male jogger who
frequently ran along the path.

He took a baseball bat and planned to knock him into unconsciousness and just lie down next to him. Luckily for the jogger, he didn't come
by that day and Dahmer tried to suppress the thoughts again.

*Physical and emotional abandonment were themes that ran through
Dahmer's entire life.* This condition strongly suggests that Dahmer, in addition to demonstrating an antisocial personality, suffered from *borderline
personality disorder* as well (fear of abandonment is the central issue mak-

ing the sufferer emotionally "clingy" and demanding of others). His parents divorced when he turned 18 years-of-age. His mother received custody of both Dahmer and his brother; however, his mother and brother soon abandoned him, leaving young Jeffrey home alone. He called his father, who eventually moved back into the family home. Soon, his father would abandon Jeffrey too. This time, Dahmer moved in with his grandmother. Due to his strange behavior, she made him move into his own apartment. Then the nightmare began as he sought out his second victim after an extensive cooling off period.

3. Albert De Salvo
"The Boston Strangler"

Parenting milieu characterized by physical abuse and emotional abandonment producing petty crime and sexual addiction; father forced prostitutes to have sex with his ten-year-old son. Reportedly, he had sex with his wife up to six times daily; alleged sexual molestation of a young girl.

sexual / from an early age. [handwritten marginal note]

Before his father left and Albert's dysfunctional parents divorced, De Salvo watched as his father knocked out his mother's teeth and broke all the fingers on one of her hands. The abuse was extremely harsh on young Albert. At one point in his childhood, a farmer paid the elder De Salvo nine dollars for Albert and two of his sisters. They escaped after a month of being slaves to the farmer. Due to his father's coaxing, when Albert was about six years old, he began petty shoplifting, which led to breaking and entering and burglary.

As Albert grew older, his father brought home prostitutes and forced Albert to watch him having sexual intercourse with them. By the age of ten, Albert had already had his first sexual experience, leading to sexual obsession. He became addicted to sex. According to reports, De Salvo claimed to have sex with his wife up to six times a day.

Later, De Salvo was dishonorably discharged from the Army due to an allegation that he sexually molested a nine-year-old girl. No conviction was obtained due to the mother's failure to file charges against him.

4. Harvey Glatman
"Lonely Hearts Killer"

Parenting milieu produced a sadomasochistic, autoerotic asphyxia addict with sexually perverted impulses.

As a child, Harvey Glatman was perceived to be "a little strange" even by the standards of his own dysfunctional parents. At the age of four, he was caught in a sadomasochistic act by inflicting pain upon himself. In the sexualized sadomasochistic act, he tied a string around his penis and the other end of the string to a drawer. He leaned back against the string, pulling it taut causing pain, and enjoying self-punishment.

Sadomasochism is defined as a sexual disorder.

⎤ When it becomes an addiction.

The string proved to be a prescient metaphor of things to come; the string became a rope he used around his neck in an obsession with auto-erotic asphyxia as an adolescent. He tied a rope around his neck and looped the free end over a pipe or rafter. He yanked the rope with one hand and masturbated with the other. He envisioned the ropes as extensions of his arms. As a serial killer, he used rope on his victims to bind them so he could control and kill them.

Psychiatrists diagnosed him with psychopathic personality, schizophrenic type, defined as "sexually perverted impulses."

5. Richard Ramirez "The Night Stalker"

Mentor was a pot-addicted killer and rapist who filled his mind with vivid images of rape and killing.

Like all serial predators, Richard Ramirez did not have a normal or peaceful childhood. Ramirez's uncle, a mentor to young Richard, was a heavy pot smoker and Vietnam veteran. He bragged to young Richard about his brutalities and sexual conquest of women during the war. He showed him many Polaroid snapshots of rape and killing; he also taught young Richard how to kill and fight.

With Ramirez present, his uncle shot his wife in the face following an argument.

6. Arthur Shawcross

Parenting milieu characterized by being sodomized with a broomstick, oral sex fetish, and incest.

Arthur Shawcross's mother was an extremely sick individual. As a child she sodomized him with a broomstick. He was told to have oral sex with his aunt, who taught him how to do it. From this experience, he adopted a fetish for oral sex. As a child he was caught having sex with his sister, an allegation his sister denies. In another instance, he was caught by his girlfriend's brother performing oral sex on her; on condition the brother kept quiet, he demanded Shawcross performed oral sex on him, his first homosexual encounter. Until age eight, Shawcross was a chronic bed wetter.

In his youth, Shawcross was a loner and never really had any friends. Growing up, he became more and more violent and this is when he began to break into houses and buildings. He became more withdrawn from the world. At the age of fourteen, he began to have oral sex with his cousin and sister.

■ Violence & Lack of "Contact Comfort"

Experimental psychologists Harry Harlow & Margaret Harlow began a series of studies in the 1950s showing the importance of **tactile stimulation** (touch) in normal behavior. The famous "contact comfort" studies extended into the mid-1960s at the University of Wisconsin and provided the first experimental evidence that *inattentive and dysfunctional mothering resulted in abnormal behavior and abnormal brain development.* Moreover, inattentive and loveless mothering "set up" (conditioned) in the offspring the propensity for some *forms of violence* later in life.

One aspect of antisocial parenting is inattentive, unaffectionate, and loveless mothering and/or fathering, producing an emotional detachment from family milieu. As mentioned previously, *milieu* is defined as important social contexts of learning (such as the home and peer groups) that emphasize *emotional connection and emotional development.*

Accordingly, Winnicott (1965) contends there is no such thing as an infant per se, meaning of course, that maternal care given the infant forms a subunit of milieu; hence mother and child are emotionally inseparable. (As the child matures, healthy development allows this natural bond to be broken; otherwise, the child experiences excessive "separation anxiety" from the mother.)

Touch
Motion
Activity

■ Monkey-ing Around

In the Harlow study, infant rhesus monkeys were chosen as subjects because, like human infants, they require long periods of *emotional attachment to caregivers,* observed in *bonding.* At birth, the experimenters isolated the infants in solitary cages where touch of any kind, attachment, or social bonding was prevented from occurring with the other monkeys.

As adults, infants *raised in isolation* were singularly withdrawn. They engaged in *self-mutating behavior* (pinching and biting themselves). Later, they channeled self-aggression into hostility—"acting out" inappropriately—against others. Infant monkeys who became adult mothers, were "brutal, indifferent mothers" to offspring. Similarly, male and female monkeys raised in isolation grew up to be "unstable, brutal" parents. *Could these results be an early parental blueprint for raising sexual psychopaths?*

■ Surrogate Mothers

In a related experiment, a group of newborn infant rhesus monkeys were placed in a cage with **surrogate** "mothers" to further test the mothering process. One "mother" was constructed of wire mesh and contained a heating lamp and a bottle with a nipple and bottle for nourishment. The other "mother" was covered in soft terrycloth with no further accoutrements (no lamp or bottle).

Under a variety of conditions (such as being frightened by a loud noise), the infants routinely chose the terrycloth-covered "mother." Even when hungry, the infants would cling to the cloth-covered "mother" while reaching across the wire "mother" for milk. The importance of *contact comfort* in the *bonding experience* between infants and mothers was experimentally verified. Prior to the Harlow's study, the *cupboard theory of attachment*—the view that infants bonded with their mothers due to the mother providing nourishment—was the dominant theory of parent-to-child bonding.

With the Harlow results, *touch and cuddling* became a significant factor in maternal and social bonding, producing healthy, well-adjusted children.

◼ Rocking: The "Nutrient" of Motion

Additionally, when the wire surrogate "mother" was replaced with a cloth-covered surrogate capable of a rocking motion, the infant monkeys *preferred the sensation of being rocked* to the motionless terrycloth surrogate. Later, as young "children," the rhesus monkeys raised with motionless cloth surrogates showed repetitive rocking movements. The monkeys who were raised with the surrogate (capable of rocking) did not display abnormal rocking movements.

Today, due to the classic study by Harlow and others, neuropsychologists are convinced that *sensory stimulation* of the variety researched by the Harlows—*holding, touching, cuddling, and rocking, or (HTCR)*—before two years of age is *necessary for normal brain development*. When one or more of the *(HTCR)* "nutrients" is lacking, irreversible, neurological deficits may occur. (Brain imaging "tools" are charting areas of the brain hit hardest by the neglect and the loveless milieu of antisocial parenting.)

Truly, the rocking chair may be the best neuropsych "tool" ever invented for development of normal brains! *Sensory enrichment* through *HTCR* leads to changes in the branching of neurons, and ion conductance, which lie at the heart of normal synaptic connectivity.

The developing brain depends on sensory stimulation to the extent that some researchers refer to touch as a "nutrient."

Shore (1996) contends . . . "infants' early emotional experiences in relation to the primary caregiver actually influence the production of certain brain chemicals that play a role in the physical development of the cortex, the part of our brain that is responsible for our most sophisticated and complex functions such as thinking, perception, and emotion. When the emotional attachment of the infant to the caregiver is stressful and unsatisfying, the hormones created in the infant's nervous system cause the abnormal development of specific structures and circuits in the cortex of the brain that are responsible for regulating emotional reactions; this abnormal brain development, triggered by negative environmental factors during the critical growth period of birth to two years of age, creates an enduring *susceptibility to various psychological disorders* later in life."

■ Advanced Attachment Theory

In 1951, British psychoanalyst John Bowlby added a human touch to the Harlow findings in rhesus monkeys when he began a series of studies of homeless children in postwar Europe. He analyzed the mother-infant bonding process leading to his *attachment theory* of bonding. That social bonding is *genetically determined* and is central to normal development of self, personality, and behavior can be analyzed according to further enhancement of his studies with the following bonding types:

1. "Type B" bonding is known as *securely attached*. Infants received optimal and consistent responsiveness from caregivers and were routinely comforted by parents in times of distress. "Type B" children displayed considerable positive affect (emotions) and resiliency.
2. Type "A" *avoidant attachment* is associated with "maternal insensitivity to infant's cues." Infants learn to "distrust parental affection as a defense against being overwhelmed by fear or sadness." "Type A" children tend to "anticipate rejection and become hostile or angry." They show less resilience in times of distress.
3. Type "C" *ambivalent/resistant attachment* with "unpredictability of emotional attachment," children become "impulsive and helpless." Although normal children, they tend to be "clingy" and insecure.
4. Type "D" *disorganized attachment* where parents become "frightening to the child" because of their own traumatic issues. Instead of providing security, parents "become an elicitor of fear." Children display "anxiety, hostility, and anger."

[handwritten margin notes: "well adjusted happy child."; "self medication through drugs / petty criminal."; "in therapy w/ low self-esteem"; "Severe extreme psychopath."]

According to researchers, Type "B"—securely attached, and Type "C"—ambivalent/resistant attachment above, fall within what is considered "normal range" without *pathological implication*.

While Type "A"—avoidant attachment—produces *difficult children* who may require professional counseling later in life, Type "D" is the *prototype for the development of the criminal mind and psychopathy*.

■ Psychology of Movement—The Cerebellum: "Nutrients" of Holding, Touching, Cuddling, & Rocking

The *cerebellum*, the three-lobed cerebral tissue behind the occipital lobe of the brain, coordinates balance and fine muscle movements. (When an inebriated person fails a field sobriety test, it's the cerebellum that nails him! Flunking the test of normal balance and coordination means the cerebellum was anesthetized due to the effects of alcohol or other drugs.)

Not surprisingly, the cerebellum is the brain center most targeted when infants and small children experience *sensory enrichment* through holding, touching, cuddling, and rocking. The author believes, somewhat "tongue-in-cheek", that an acid test for whether or not a given child is receiving adequate HTCR is for Mom or Dad to playfully throw their three-year-old child up the air (not too far!) as most parents are prone to do in play. If the child's eyes widen in fear, getting stiff from head to toe, the implication is that the brain's motion center—the cerebellum—is somewhat dissonant to HTCR (unless this was the first time to be tossed up in the air). If the child gleefully smiles and says, "Do it again!", we have some **anecdotal** evidence that the cerebellum is becoming finely tuned due to the enhanced development attributable to HTCR. As any parent knows, children who are playfully thrown in the air and caught love it. According to the author's experience, when this occurs outside in the front yard in plain view of other children, a "me next" line soon forms. The same rationale holds true for swinging, sliding, jumping on a trampoline, riding a bike, or riding on the merry-go-round.

Kids love motion—running, jumping, spinning around and falling down. Apparently, the brain requires motion for normal development. In a practical and beneficial way, youth sports enhance early (before age two) parent-child interactive play. Non-contact sports such as gymnastics, swimming, tennis, and, to a lesser extent, soccer and volleyball seem especially beneficial. Due to the likelihood of head trauma, the physical violence of football, rugby, and boxing can exacerbate pre-existing neurological damage with vicious blows to the head (e.g. currently observed in the violent, social behavior of Mike Tyson, and the nearly incomprehensible verbiage of former professional boxers Joe Frazier, Muhammad Ali, and Michael Spinks). Some authorities believe the cumulative effects of the "head butt" in soccer and volleyball can lead to blunt head trauma.

According to brain neuroscientist Dr. James Prescott (of the *National Institute of Child Health and Human Development*) "when touch and movement receptors and their projections to other brain structures do not receive *sufficient sensory stimulation*, normal development and function" (does not occur). Dr. Prescott believes the cerebellum is involved in *complex emotional behavior* so that under-stimulation can have devastating effects upon *emotionality* later in life.

Relative to "complex emotional behavior", we now turn to one of the most despised serial killers in history with the Predator Profile of the "killer clown" John Wayne Gacy.

PREDATOR PROFILE (6-1)

John Wayne Gacy
"The Killer Clown"

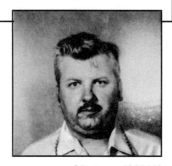

Span of Time Crimes Committed:

1972–1978

Physical Description of Offender:

White Male
5' 9" Tall
Grey Hair
Blue Eyes
Weight 215 lbs.
DOB 3-17-42

Offenses Prior to Serial Killing:

In 1969, Gacy was convicted of sodomy of a teenage male, for which he served three years of a ten-year sentence in a State of Iowa correctional facility.

Victimology:

Type of victims selected: homosexual or heterosexual males (early teens into late twenties). Ostensibly, Gacy lured victims to his home with promise of drugs, sex, or employment. Often, he *impersonated a police officer*, making his victims think they were being arrested. Once victims were in Gacy's car or in his home, he used chloroform to disorient and sedate them. He proceeded to torture, rape, and kill his victims by strangulation. A necrophiliac, Gacy had sex with victims after they were deceased. Gacy buried all but four victims under the crawlspace in his home.

Current Status:

Gacy was executed on May 10, 1994.

Comments:

To the casual observer in everyday life, Gacy appeared to be a normal person. He was a well-regarded and respected individual in the community. He was successful in business as a construction contractor. In a macabre twist, he volunteered at local hospitals as *Pogo the Clown* to entertain children. Friends and business associates never suspected Gacy's narcissistic proclivities that masked the serial killer just beneath his civic persona.

The types of crimes Gacy committed coincide with an *organized* type of killer. Gacy was well prepared for his victims by keeping items to drug and/or restrain them in his home and vehicle. Gacy used alcohol and drugs to heighten feeling while committing the crimes. He left enough time after his crimes to clean up before his wife and children came home. Therefore, he chose victims close to home.

Student Contributors:

Stacy Arnett and Jack Shannon

STUDENT ANAYLSIS: *The Psychopathy of John Wayne Gacy*

John Wayne Gacy was a vicious serial killer who preyed on young males from the early to late 1970s. *Gacy was convicted of thirty-three murders.* How many others he committed authorities will never know.

Gacy grew up in a strict, Catholic family with an abusive alcoholic father. Gacy was married twice; however his first wife divorced him when he was sent to prison for sodomy of a male teenager. Gacy served three years of a ten-year sentence for that crime in the State of Iowa. Prison reformers ask "why only three years?" While he was in prison his father passed away, distressing Gacy. Being incarcerated was just another way of disappointing his father, whom he felt he could never please.

Once released from prison, Gacy moved to Chicago and began living a seemingly normal life—on the surface. Gacy became a self-employed construction contractor and a high profile member of the local chapter of the Jaycees. He was soon elected as president of the civic organization. Gacy was well known for throwing lavish parties for his friends and business associates. He was known as *Pogo the Clown* and appearing in local hospitals in his clown suit and painted face to entertain children.

Gacy married a woman he had known in high school named Carol Huff. She was divorced with two daughters of her own. While dating her and before they married, Gacy confided in her that he considered himself bisexual. After a few months of marriage, Gacy's wife learned of his addiction to pornography. He compulsively masturbated, watching his porno, instead of having sex with his wife.

The strange smell coming from under the house bothered his wife even more. In a short time, she filed for divorce and left him. Strangely, they remained friends after the divorce.

The police tied Gacy to the disappearance of his last victim, Robert Piest, due to the fact Piest told his mother he would be home after his job interview with Gacy. Unfortunately, Piest never made it home. Authorities checked Gacy's criminal history and discovered Gacy had been accused of several attacks on homosexual men, but the allegations had never been proven. They obtained a search warrant to search Gacy's residence for any evidence of Piest. At the time, they failed to locate any evidence, but suspicion remained. They placed Gacy under surveillance. A second search was initiated shortly thereafter. This time, they checked the crawlspace under his home, which revealed what Gacy later called "my own personal cemetery." Police recovered 29 bodies from under the house and four more from the river.

Student Contributor:

Stacy Arnett, criminal profiling student

◼ Displeasure Centers

Once known as physiological psychologists (and later psychobiologists), **neuroscientists** study the effects of early environmental influences on behavior, and therefore, on the brain. Since the mid-1960s, researchers have known that mere external electrode stimulation of the anterior hypothalamus (within the limbic system) produced violent behavior. Dr. James Olds, a trailblazer in electrode stimulation of the brain, discovered "pleasure centers" in the **medial forebrain bundle (MFB)** of the hypothalamus. (In self-stimulation studies, a rat will level-press up to 5,000 times in one hour when the electrode passes through the MFB, a center rich in the neurotransmitter dopamine.) Not far away, Olds discovered a "displeasure" center near the hypothalamus and associated areas known as the amygdala.

Does lack of motion (and HTCR) in infancy and young childhood contribute to the emotion of displeasure, and perhaps "acting-out" behavior later in childhood? As early as 1975, Dr. Robert Heath of Tulane University showed that the emotional centers of the brain's *limbic system* (specifically the **hippocampus**, amygdala, and **septal areas**) did interconnect with the cerebellum.

According to Dr. Heath "... violence may result from a *permanent defect in the pleasure centers* (due to) inadequate early mothering. The infant who is deprived of movement and physical closeness will fail to develop the brain pathways that mediate pleasure ... such people may be suffering at the neuronal level from *stunted growth of the pleasure system.*"

Anhedonia

In Dr. Heath's view, due to a scarcity of cell connection, the expression of pleasure is not "broadcast" properly throughout the brain. The immature cerebellum develops abnormally in infants and young children deprived of HTCR. Fewer connections (reflects low activity) between the cerebellum and pleasure centers may result in a condition known as **anhedonia**—decreased ability to feel pleasure—which may produce an insatiable desire to experience pleasure. In the absence of pleasure, frustration and anger may be experienced where "acting out" violently occurs as an attempt to experience some measure of pleasure.

Apparently, neuronal connections required to experience sustained feelings of pleasure were not "hard-wired" in the brain at developmentally significant times. The developmental timeframe is theorized to be before age three.

Might the "red flags" associated with the developing psychopathy—cruelty to pets, setting fires, fighting, and anger outbursts—occur due to the frustration of not feeling pleasure and *to low amplitude or inactivity* in cerebral neurons?

Interestingly, psychiatric patients at Tulane University Medical School treated with *cerebellar stimulation*—internal stimulation of the cerebellum—reported nearly miraculous results. A "pacemaker technique" of stimulation produced a decrease of emotional outbursts. Might this be an effective way to at least partially reverse a history of HTCR deprivation in young children? Could this treatment derail some of the neurological damage observed in psychopathy? Does enough funding exist to continue the studies?

▪ Eriksonian Developmental Theory— Implications in Psychopathy

Early Childhood Stage (Ages 6 to 7 years)

Salient aspects of Erik Erikson's developmental stage theory of psychosocial "crises," selected for relevancy, will be presented as a template over which elements of antisocial parenting can be observed.

Underlying curricula in many nursing programs in North America and much of the world, Erikson's *psychosocial developmental theory* recognizes a series of *emotional crises* that must be addressed at sequential stages. When successfully resolved, individuals leave the stage *emotionally enhanced.* They move to the next stage *with a positive emotional experience* to build upon. When unsuccessfully resolved, individuals *suffer emotional deficits* (as well as neurological glitches) entering subsequent stages; they move on with less emotional stamina, resilience, and neurological functioning.

safe feelings.

With success, growth and emotion slowly build one upon the other. The emotional "crises" are resolved with effective, nurturing experiences. Children enter each succeeding stage emotionally robust. Fragile self-esteem is nurtured along the way. However, deficits experienced in earlier stages tend to sabotage succeeding stages. When emotional needs are not being actualized, children often display behavioral "red flags" associated with oppositional defiant behavior.

It is instructive to locate the "acting out" behavior observed in **ODD (Oppositional defiant disorder)** at one end of a deviancy continuum while observing the withdrawn, brooding, and reclusive behavior characterized by the **schizotypal personality disorder** at the other pole. Both abnormal behavioral types—*oppositional defiant and schizotypal*—characterize potential criminal behavior. As personality studies demonstrate, oppositional defiant category of deviance gravitates toward violence and psychopathy.

Trust versus Mistrust—Implications in Psychopathy

Erikson believes the *infancy stage* (birth to first year of life) produces the first emotional crisis needing resolution as *trust versus mistrust.* This initial stage acts as the foundation on which all other stages are constructed.

Care, nurturing, parental attentiveness and competence in meeting infants' needs prepare the child to trust caregivers. The emotional benchmark of trust acts as buoyancy to budding self-esteem, as infants move into Stage Two (second year of life). In this stage, effective *toilet training strategies* produce a sense of *autonomy* versus an overly demanding or impatient training regime that translates as internalized feelings of shame and/or doubt. (Freud theorized "anal retentive" personality characteristics erupted at this stage producing *obsessive-compulsive* behavior leading to OCD, or obsessive-compulsive disorder, later in life.)

Third year through fifth year of life produces the *play stage* and a crisis of *initiative* versus guilt. The very essence of *motivation* may arise in this critical stage. *Sequencing of behavior,* where children learn "what comes next" subsequent to termination of events such as play, study, eating, or sleeping, arise in this stage. Smart, involved parents teach children to pick up toys, get homework done before TV, and keep their rooms organized and clean—all strategies considered normal. Otherwise, parents are promoting **learned helplessness** in their children who often live like "slobs" in unkempt bedrooms or apartments.

It is easy to see how unfulfilled emotional crises start to implode around the increasing dysfunctional life of the developing psychopath. In antisocial parenting—by age five—trust, autonomy, and initiative have been systemically replaced as parents have failed their children by promoting *mistrust, shame, doubt, and guilt.* As emotional abusive and hateful parenting increases, it is not surprising to discover the start of oppositional defiant behavior in preteens. In none of the first three stages of development has the child felt loved or valued.

Stage Four (ages six through puberty) sets up a crisis of *industry versus inferiority.* Loving and competent parents who display nurturing, attention, and care for children produce a sense of achievement and productivity (industry) with the successful resolution of this stage. Normal children gain a *sense of purpose.* On the other hand, antisocial parenting produces frustration, anger, and emotional deviance as dominant feelings. The child is consumed with feelings of inferiority.

Incarcerated criminals often discuss feeling "inferior" or "powerless" as the motivation to commit serial crimes. The same motivation extends into "Rambo" adolescent killers.

■ The Central Importance of Mothering

Many developmental psychologists believe that the most important adult figure in early childhood development (up to age three) is the mother. A sense of belonging and love (or lack of) appears to be a strong *emotional sentiment* developed during this time. Evidence from incarceration interviews with serial offenders shows the relationship with antisocial mothering was uniformly *cool, distant, unloving, and neglectful,* characterized by a lack of *emotional warmth.* Infants who eventually grew up to become serial killers *never internalized maternal love* from an early age. Internalizing abuse—sexual, verbal, mental, and/or physical—continually showed up in interviews with serial killers.

Growing up with an emotionally absent mother, and often a literally absent father, it is no wonder children grow up angry and oppositional defiant. They have received practically no behavioral limits, or by contrast, nearly intolerable boundaries. This condition produced a nihilistic "monster" incapable of caring for and nurturing others.

◼ Deviant Egocentric Mindset

Comprehending the world in *egocentric* ways characterizes the early developmental stages of childhood development in both normal and psychopathic children. However, as normal children develop, they become less egocentric and more empathetic. They can see the world from another's perspective. By contrast, the psychopath becomes more egocentric. He often hides his fragile ego behind arrogance and inflated confidence. Listen to the way he talks about himself; it always gives him away.

The renowned Swiss developmental psychologist, Jean Piaget (1896–1980) demonstrated egocentricity with his famous "Three Mountains" experiment. Children were seated across a small table from a doll and were asked to judge a papier-mache model of three mountains, as it would appear from the doll's perspective. The responses were selected from a number of cards depicting different angles of the mountains in relation to the different perspectives around the table. Pre-operational children (ages two to seven) chose the picture of the mountain *from their own perspective,* not the doll's perspective, an example of egocentric thinking. In contrast, the older, concrete operational children (ages seven to twelve) most often chose the correct picture, the way the mountains looked from the doll's side of the table (Piaget and Inhelder, 1956). Metaphorically, adolescent psychopaths have the same egocentricity of pre-operational children. Life is all about them.

As deviance grows in the concrete operational child (ages seven–twelve), it would be interesting to test Piaget's research on the neurologically damaged brain of the "developing" psychopath. We suspect the psychopathic child to visually choose the correct angle due to his age, yet emotional immaturity would be highly visible.

The lethal combination of *superficial normalcy* observed in many psychopaths, paired with *emotional immaturity and egocentricity,* with increasing focus on *sexual perversity,* explains why sexual psychopaths (serial killers) are so dangerous to unsuspecting victims.

Strong, influential adult role models never emerge in the first seven years of life in the slowly "simmering" development of psychopathic personality. Interestingly, Freud theorized that much of personality is "set" by age six or seven and becomes highly resistant to change, a view that reinforces the *irreversibility* of psychopathy.

◼ Childhood Stage (ages eight–twelve years)—Implications in Psychopathy

In a child entering puberty, a boy needs a strong, stabilizing figure in his life; boys need a loving father. More than half (over 18 of the original 36 respondents) of all serial killers studied saw their fathers leave the home during this stage. Absent fathers produce anger, embarrassment, and worst of all *loneliness* during this stage. Feeling *isolated* and *lonely* characterizes a salient feature of psychopathy from lifelong *emotional scarcity*.

Also damaging is the fact that preadolescent sexuality and fantasies are not connected to another person; rather they emerge as *autoerotic, rape fantasies* (at approximately 12 to 14 years of age). Perverse fantasies may be exacerbated by a pronounced fascination with pornography, fetishism, voyeurism, and compulsive masturbation in mid-to-late adolescence. Entering adolescence, both garden variety and sexual psychopaths are immature and socially incompetent; that is, they lack the social skills required to foster normal interpersonal relationships. They have many short-term relationships that end according to their egocentric view because of "the other person."

Launched from this developmental stage feeling inferior, some "becoming" psychopaths remain painfully introverted and shy (Edmund Kemper types), but some appear extraverted with a "gift of gab" (Ted Bundy types), masking their inner loneliness, deviance, and emotional desperation.

Deviant Sexual Fantasies

Deviant sexual fantasies spill over into the mind of adolescents on the brink of entering adult sexuality, yet they are far from feeling like proactive, independent adults. Deviant sexualized fantasies further erode any hope of developing normal social and sexual skills with consenting adults, so that resentment for not having nurturing experiences from competent parenting further exacerbates oppositional defiance.

According to Ressler, loneliness, isolation, and sexual "daydreaming" provide an emotional platform for cruelty to animals and other children, truancy, setting fires, fighting, and assaulting teachers. Later, as young adults, they are unstable in the workplace as job "hoppers," and underachievers in school, further evidence of their greatest fear that others will discover their incompetence and inferiority feelings. Later adolescence (14 to 18 years of age) produces compulsive masturbation, lying, promiscuous sex, and nightmares. Adolescent psychopaths sleep very poorly and wake up chronically tired.

Entering young adulthood, the possibility of acting out deviant fantasies becomes an obsession. The world is perceived as a cruel place. With little restraint on oppositional deviant behavior in middle childhood, sexual themes of dominance, molestation, manipulation, and revenge fuels aggression and the need to "act out." As the teen years transcend into young adulthood, time draws near to unleash rapacious behavior on "deserving" victims.

The nihilistic and egocentric mindset of rapists and murderers allows them to *depersonalize* victims as "objects" to fulfill sexual fantasies. Deviant cognitive maps set up neural pathways in the brain with tainted, sadistic, and rapacious sexuality.

Stressors (or environmental "triggers") provide the final push into rapacious behavior—preying on others. The loss of a job, a relationship breakup, or financial problems triggers the actualization of deviant fantasies. The "straw that broke the camel's back" can be something minor in relation to what normal people adjust to in everyday life.

Magical thinking enters the mindset of human predators diagnosed with paranoid schizophrenics, a severe thought disorder. For example, serial killer Richard Chase, the "Vampire Killer," believed his own blood would "magically" turn to powder if he did not drink the blood of his victims. Yet, as we have shown, the vast majority of serial predators are not mentally ill; they know exactly what they're doing. What's more, they're compelled to keep doing it.

◼ Adolescent Stage (ages 12–18)— Implications in Psychopathy

The crisis of *identity* versus *role confusion* characterizes this stage of development as personality becomes more integrated (or less integrated) as peer pressure and parental expectations remain highly influential.

Inside the mind of the young psychopath, what identity resides? Speculative logic dictates *role confusion,* isolation, frustration, anger, and egocentricity. Dave Berkowitz, "The Son of Sam," was an accomplished fire-starter before his "career" as a serial killer.

PREDATOR PROFILE (6-2)

David Berkowitz
"The Son of Sam"

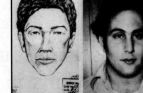
©Bettmann/CORBIS

Alternative Media Moniker:

"The .44 Caliber Killer"

Time Span Crimes Committed:

New York, July 29, 1976 until July 31,1977

Physical Description of Killer:

Of Jewish heritage, Berkowitz was approximately 5 feet 6 inches tall, small framed, and short black curly hair.

Offenses Prior to Killing:

By his own documentation, he set 1,488 fires in New York. He had three counts of attempted murder by stabbing three women, all of whom survived. He wanted media recognition for the crimes; when media failed to recognize him, the serial murders began.

Berkowitz stalked women who were parked in cars alone or sitting with friends. All of the female victims were in their late teens to mid-twenties. He killed them with a Bulldog .44 pistol.

Current Status:

He is forty-nine years of age and serving 365 years. Formerly at Attica Correctional Facility, he is currently a resident at Sullivan Correctional Facility, Fallsburg, NY.

General Comments:

David's mother, Betty, could not afford to take care of him and gave him up for adoption. Nat and Pearl Berkowitz adopted him at an early age. Berkowitz grew up in the Bronx, NY, and had a relatively normal childhood. He was mostly introverted and self-conscious about his appearance because he was physically larger than his peers. Neighbors saw David as a bully who did not get along well with others. He was hyperactive and difficult to control at times.

When Berkowitz was fourteen, his adoptive mother, Pearl, died from breast cancer in 1967. After her death, he adopted a negative attitude that affected his grades and behavior. Nat remarried a woman who was not fond of Berkowitz. His adoptive father moved to Florida to be with his wife. Berkowitz thought Pearl's death and his abandonment was out of spite to destroy him. It was during this time he sought to live in his own fantasy world.

Berkowitz joined the army in 1971. His desire was to be a hero and gain recognition. He was an excellent marksman with a rifle. Berkowitz had one sexual experience with a woman in Korea and contracted a venereal disease. He left the army in 1974 and began a quest to find his biological mother. David found his mother and his sister, Roslyn.

He attempted to reunite with them as a family. Eventually, David became bored with this effort. He failed to keep in contact with his mother and sister.

Shortly after, he started setting fires in New York and kept a journal listing each one. Authorities suspect this behavior was an effort to gain control of his life. He had always wanted to be a fireman, but he never took the qualifying test. He felt emotionally stimulated when bodies were brought out of a burning building; he fantasized about fiery plane crashes.

According to Robert Ressler, "most arsonists like the feeling that they are responsible for the excitement and violence of a fire. With the simple act of lighting matches, they control events in society that are not normally controlled—they orchestrate the fire, the screaming arrival and deployment of the fire trucks and fire fighters, the gathering crowds, the destruction of property and sometimes of people."

Berkowitz began a reclusive lifestyle, leaving his apartment only for food. He would write things on the walls . . . "In this hole lives the Wicked King. Kill for my Master. I turn children into Killers."

During this time, he claimed demons possessed him. He was under the delusion that his neighbor Sam was demonic and Sam's demons controlled his thoughts and actions, hence the title "Son of Sam." David maintained an insanity conviction after he was caught. He claimed that Sam's demon-possessed dog instructed him to kill others. That plan was transparent to FBI profiler Robert Ressler. Later, Berkowitz admitted the "dog story" was a hoax.

The "demons" and the resentment at his mother for dying and abandonment led him on a killing spree. On July 29, 1976, David shot and killed 18-year-old Donna Lauria. Later, David said that he killed Donna to please "Sam and the demons."

David traveled from New York to Texas to purchase both the gun and ammunition used in the murders. He felt they could not be traced.

David left behind a note at the first crime scene stating: "I say goodbye and good night. Police, let me haunt you with these words: I'll be back! I'll be back! To be interpreted as Bang, Bang, Bang, Bang, Bang-Ugh!! Yours in murder, Mr. Monster." Ironically, Berkowitz fired five shots equivalent to the amount of "bangs" used in the note. He almost always fired five shots during his murders.

From July 29, 1976 until July 31, 1977 David killed six people and injured six others using his .44 caliber pistol. He stalked women nightly, anticipating the location of each murder. If he could not find someone worthy enough to kill he would revisit one of the previous crime scenes, become sexually aroused, and masturbate. Killing the women justified his anger and aroused him at the same time.

Upon capture, he expressed the desire after some of the killings to attend victims' funerals, but abstained from going out of fear of police guards at the ceremonies. He wanted to know if the media was paying attention to his murder spree. Often, he hung around diners listening to conversations among people or even officers to note whether or not his crimes had become public.

During his killings, Berkowitz began corresponding with newspaper columnist Jimmy Breslin. The columnist printed expanded accounts of the Son of Sam killings, which may have enticed him to kill more. He loved attention. Authorities have argued that Breslin was indirectly responsible for the continuation of the Son of Sam murders.

Berkowitz was captured on August 10, 1977. He was quoted saying that he "wanted to go out in a blaze of glory." Clinicians diagnosed Berkowitz as a paranoid schizophrenic. As inmate, he kept a scrapbook of newspaper articles about his crimes.

Berkowitz had a standard parole hearing on July 9, 2002. As an inmate, he converted to Christianity. He has worked as the chaplain's clerk. He says he does not deserve parole. At the time of the murders he characterized his mood as "tormented in mind or spirit."

Complied and Edited by:

Heather Kidd, criminal profiling student

Aftermath

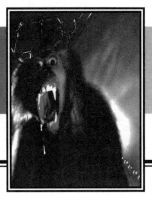

I. Word Scholar

Define the following words from *The Word Scholar Glossary*.

1. Toxic parenting _____

2. Tactile stimulation _____

3. Anhedonia _____

4. Learned helplessness _____

5. Magical thinking _____

6. Autoerotic asphyxia _____

7. Sadomasochism _____

8. HTCR "nutrients" _____

9. Medial Forebrain Bundle (MFB) _____

10. Oppositional Defiant Disorder (ODD) _____

II. The Forensic Lab

Compose a one page report addressing: A strong argument (like you would make in court as a forensic neuropsychologist) that parents should be held criminally liable for the violence perpetrated upon others by their underage adolescent children. Why not? What prevented them from seeking competent psychiatric help? Is there any valid excuse?

CHAPTER 7

The Psychology of Perversion: Adolescent "Rambo" Killers & Female Serial Killers

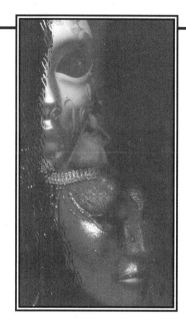

66 . . . *When she bent to look, he brought the plaster cast down on the back of her head . . . (after) a succession of blows, none of them too hard, she slumped over the chair . . . He slit the blouse up the back with a pair of bandage scissors, pulled the blouse off, and handcuffed her hands behind her . . . 'Good,' he said.* **99**

—*Silence of the Lambs*
Thomas Harris

"Child abuse or neglect, unstable or erratic parenting, or inconsistent parental discipline may increase the likelihood that Conduct Disorder will evolve into Antisocial Personality Disorder."

—DSM-IV-TR

This chapter, the *psychology of perversion,* focuses on the behavior of women and children who become perpetrators of violence. Kids, many too young to drive, are kids who kill other kids and adults in homeplace and schoolplace violence—adolescent "Rambo" killers—in our nomenclature. The remainder of the chapter provides an overview of Females Who Kill, such as "Black Widows" and "Angels of Death".

The slow metamorphosis from normalcy to perversion is a by-product of horrific parenting—*antisocial parenting*—producing deep emotional scars that "rewire" the brain toward violence, producing individuals so neurologically damaged and behaviorally perverted we believe the word "sapient" (wise) no longer applies. As previously noted, we suggest *pseudo-sapien* is more descriptive of a human predator—a person with reptilian appetites.

Although abused and mistreated, small children, screaming and crying, cling to incompetent "caregivers" when parents are arrested in their
presence and taken from the home. "Please don't put my Daddy in jail,"
one child lamented, "who's going to take *care of me?*" To the child, "care"
may be the only word he or she knows, but to CPS (child protective service) and police investigators, "care" is defined as incompetence, neglect,
and abuse. Authorities know where these kids are headed. They know
every single social agency is going to fail them. Young girls may end up in
depressing *co-dependency* relationships, or as drug addicted prostitutes. In
her self-hatred she may turn to petty crime or she may become a killer.
Often, the boys become violent criminals and/or sexual psychopaths, the
serial killers of society.

> *Psychopathy starts in the home but the predictable outcome—vio-
> lence—ends in many places and has many faces.*

Due to hateful antisocial parenting, normal development of the brain
is rendered perverted and abnormal. The extent of the trauma is being
documented by brain scanning technology showing "cool-coded" blue
(denoting minimal blood flow and activity). Psychopathy "hides" in cerebral tissues known as the temporal lobes, cerebellum, amygdala, and the
prefrontal lobes—the center for restraint, behavioral and social appropriateness and "end result" consequences—behavior blatantly absent in sexual psychopathy.

Soon, sophisticated brain scanning will continually evolve to show
clear demarcation between normalcy and abnormality in neural centers.
The brains of kids in primary school with propensity to kill their classmates will be shown to be neurologically different. We predict these sophisticated brain scans will show a decreased networking of "restraint centers"
that "broadcast" to prefrontal lobes and associated cortices via thalamus
and other neural pathways. With restraint muted, what do we expect?

We can envision a time in the near future, unless all schools are
equipped with metal detectors, besides a vaccine record children will have
to show evidence of brain scans before they are allowed to register for
public schools. "Cool-coded" scans, showing damaged prefrontal lobes,
will send those children off to clinical facilities.

In the meantime, the *preponderance of the evidence*—the very weight
of all that neuroscience and experimental psychology knows about human
development, cognition, and affective (emotional) centers in the brain
and how this knowledge stacks up against sexualized perversion, violence,
and deviant cognitive mapping—is far too consequential to ignore. We
have classic, long-standing animal studies both in North America and the
UK with decades of replication in labs around the world documenting the
neuropsychological ramifications of touch, bonding, cognitive mapping,
and cerebellar inactivity pointing to neurological damage and psychopathy. And, now we have brain scans.

◼ "Cool-Coded" Brain Scans—Prefrontal Lobe Damage

Now, with forensic neuroscience and brain scanning technology squarely in the courtroom showing telltale "cool-coded" blue of *prefrontal lobe damage* in human predators, evidence for "the why" of sexual psychopathy, while shocking, is no longer mysterious. At least we have a reason why their behavior is unstable and violent. We understand why they are serial killers.

Forensic neuroscientists are showing jurors the cause of sexual psychopathy with "cool-coded" blue areas of inactivity in brain scans. In most cases, the juries are swayed by it.

Juries are agreeing with science and mitigating first-degree murder—showing premeditation and a mind clear of pathology—to second-degree murder and life in prison, often without the possibility of parole. (In the process, taxpayers (like you and me) are funding unlimited dental, medical, and educational opportunities, not to mention meals and sleeping quarters, for incarcerated criminals, many of whom are on death row for committing horrific crimes.)

This chapter addresses the deviant and perverted *psychosocial development* of emotionally damaged children and adolescents and emotionally fractured women, many of them mothers, who kill husbands, boyfriends, children in the neighborhood, and their own children.

This chapter is an **apocalyptical** wake-up call that speaks to core issues of women and children in North American society. Social historians remind us that civilizations start declining and free fall into **decadence** when mothers and children are not protected from emotional and physical abuses, or when mothers and children become so violent themselves, the very essence of the family unit is in danger of becoming breeding grounds for violence and psychopathy. Until families learn to be competent, skillful, loving, and respectful of human dignity, and schools become empowered with **in loco parentis** to do their jobs with authority, it will only get worse. Netherworld will become Huxley's brave new world.

Getting caught "red-handed" by authorities in schools or in homes by shocked parents is the only reason "Rambo" killers do not progress into the ranks of serial killers. The most shocking statistic is how young they are—eleven to eighteen-years-of-age!

◼ *Sui Generis* Classification— Pseudo-Sapien "Rambo" Killers

"Rambo" killers reside somewhere along the psychopathic continuum with serial killers, rapists, and other *malum in se* criminals (literally a crime "evil in itself"). "Rambo" killers ambush and kill their parents in their own homes. They bring weapons to school seeking to kill classmates, teachers, staff, janitors, and principals. Seldom showing remorse, they kill with guns, knives, baseball bats, brickbats, and bare hands. Some, like the teenagers at Columbine, go out in a blaze of suicidal glory in the context of guerilla warfare. This occurs not in some faraway country defending democracy, but in the halls of suburban high schools amid middle-to-upper-class values in decent communities.

Born and Reared in Pop Culture USA

Being captured during or shortly after they kill is the only thing that prevents "Rambo" killers from killing again. They are born of **Pop Culture USA**—the hedonistic "religion" of North America and they are nurtured by it.

It is important to understand that popular culture (*pop culture* for short) is never about *competence, morality, decency, or ethical behavior.* Pop culture is about *appearances, superficiality, hedonism, recreational drug use, and* **pseudo-intellectualism**. At best, pop culture is *pretentious, flashy,* and *seeks immediate BandAid® solutions;* at its worst, it is the harbinger of thugs, criminals, and psychopaths, masquerading as normal, everyday citizens.

Christianity and Catholicism, once moral compasses to righteous behavior, have been reduced to ritualistic **dogma**. The major religions of North America have lost out in a "tug-of-war" with pop culture hedonism. As statistics of criminal behavior pile up against wholesome morality, the evidence for failure of morality is right in our faces every time we purchase a newspaper or watch the evening news. Many citizens choose to bury their heads in the sand of denial.

■ Behaving Badly

Some priests, preachers, youth ministers, and televangelists *behaving badly* have all but driven the stake into the heart of religion as a seriously taken ideology. Recently documented examples of clergy behaving badly include child porn sites found on church computers, alter boy molestation by priests, sixteen-year-old girls or boys having sex with youth ministers, pastors having sex with the secretaries and the flock. The message from pulpits is clear: preach one thing and practice another. Put on your Sunday best. If "you look good, and you're in a good place, you must be good." Yes, we know the argument—they're just people like everyone else. Regardless, the damage done by **hypocrisy** is especially cruel to young minds lacking perspective, maturity, and experience. The attitude "we sin like everybody else, but we're saved" reeks of insincerity and impropriety. This mindset is especially dangerous to sexual psychopaths who often operate out of religious obsession. They "know" they have God's forgiveness no matter how much they "rip up" victims. They have forgiveness of a higher power.

■ Neurotheology

Using "higher centers" of the brain, a truly spiritual lifestyle requires restraint, morals, ethics, and certain amount of compulsivity in weighing consequences (see William James' *Varieties of Religious Experience,* Collier, 1966 for an excellent discussion between *religiosity* versus *spirituality*). The argument made by some **neurotheologists** is compelling. In order to combat the powerful influence of pop culture perhaps society needs less **ostentatious** religion and more profound spirituality. (Chapter Eight contains more details of the spiritual "science" of **neurotheology.**)

In contrast, "lower centers" of the brain (the reptilian and mid-brain centers) have neural centers of pleasure—places that jazz and stimulate revelers who seek **pan-hedonism**—sexuality, drugs, and the innuendo of danger in relationships. For the young and beautiful—the mannequins of pop culture, full of hopes and dreams—the message is particularly seductive. Hedonistic **aphorism** abounds: "if you look good, if you have any measure of fame, or if you make a lot of money, *you must be good.*" When a pop culture "icon"—a celebrity—is interviewed, America listens as if expecting to hear something profound (we may or we may not hear profundity). What do we expect to hear from self-centered narcissists who have embraced the very essence of pop culture as their ticket to fame? What we usually get is variations on *pseudo-intellectualism.* (If you use a big word, you must be smart. For example, how many times have you heard celebrities use the word "**epiphany**"? It's one of their favorite words.) Spending their entire lives in a career devoted to playing other people may explain why some have so much trouble "finding themselves."

Pop culture looks really good as surface shine, just don't "pop the hood" because chances are you're "buying" a lemon.

■ YAAVIST Society—The Components of Pop Culture USA

According to Jacobs (1992), the following components of pop culture (the list is by no means exhaustive) are influential in providing a launch pad for *psychological manipulation* by product manufacturers through **consumerism** in all its forms. However, it is the less recognized *psychological impact* on the minds and behavior of young adolescents and adults who have the power of transform. YAAVIST society pertains to:

1. Youth. A familiar slogan by a soft drink manufacturer states: "Think Young. Drink Pepsi." The over-40 crowd, especially middle-aged and senior-aged individuals lose out to the media blitz of fresh-faced young bodies. *Forget mind. Forget personality.* Think young, sexualized bodies. The message inflates self-importance and body-type as indicator of desirability and even success. Many young adolescents and young adults don't feel they "match" the almost unattainable visual images in magazines and in electronic media. The "Y" in YAAVIST is all about *appearances, superficiality, and physicality* as the banner headlines of pop culture. You're in the "in crowd" with them, the superficial allure, the full banquet table afforded adolescent youth.

2. Attractive. Closely related to youth, attractiveness—looking beautiful or handsome—is equated with sexuality and desirability. Reality TV

cashes in on the pop culture obsession of youth and attractiveness. The message from media advertisers is: "If you don't have it, then spend the money necessary to get it." The alternative is exclusion from YAAV-IST Society. Liposuction. Breast Enhancement. Rhinoplasty. Face-lift. Tummy Tuck. The standard for beauty in North America is practically unattainable with the airbrushed perfection of pop culture mannequin-like models. YAAVIST showcases individuals with garden variety psychopathy. For aging psychopaths and everyone else, next stop: Botox® injections and red corvettes.

3. Visual. Since visual imagery is the "language" of pop culture, we expect to be blitzed with youthful and attractive bodies and young faces. The visual message is disturbing: "if you look good, you must be good." *Trust is established at a glance.* Generally, females considered serial killer Ted Bundy somewhat attractive. Armed with a sling around his arm (hiding a crowbar), decked out in a business suit, and blessed with an engaging personality and "gift of gab," he approached females on college campuses asking help carrying books to his car. Those who complied . . . died. Some of the bodies were never found. Pop culture dazzles with visual appearances and surface shine. YAAVIST is like a low-calorie health drink, filling for the moment, but lacking substantive nutrition.

4. Isolation. Not wanting to be left out, young males and females clamor to the bars and nightclubs with hopes of finding conversation, companionship, maybe sex, and even love. Where else? Everyone wants to be an **extravert**—a people person—whether or not they naturally fit the typology. Trying to be someone they're not, they shun the label of being an **introvert** with the resulting connotation of a pathological loner, which could not be farther from the truth. The *RAS* (reticular activation system) in the brain determines the "amplitude" of incoming sensation determining the *attitudes of introversion versus extroversion.* (See *Psychology of Adjustment,* D. Jacobs (2002) for further discussion of Carl Jung's *Attitudes and Functions of Personality.*) Interviewed on death row, *serial* killers feel *isolation from mainstream interaction. They feel rejected by those they fantasize about and eventually kill.*

5. Success. Dress. Cars. Jewelry. Pop culture caters to those with money to buy whatever consumable products are perceived to keep us young, attractive, sexy, thin, and desirable. We need go no further than the billion dollar-a-year profiteers of diet schemes promising perfect bodies as the quickest way to "have our dreams come true." As everyone knows, if a person drives an expensive sports car and wears nice clothes, he or she *must be successful, therefore, desirable.*

6. Thin Body. The most recognizable image of pop culture is thin, *sexualized bodies,* the perfectly proportioned "mannequins" that youth seeks to emulate. Skipping meals, smoking cigarettes, and taking harmful "weight loss" drugs rob important vitamins and minerals from blood and tissue, causing catastrophic health problems in later life. The focus of YAAVIST is here and now. Forget tomorrow.

In conclusion, *hedonism* is the anthem of this ultimate pop culture call YAAVIST. The automotive industry, cosmetic and clothing manufacturers, perfume and cologne manufactures, vacation programs, diet plans, health clubs, and "healthy" prepackaged "nutritional" foods, all line up in TV-land, magazine ads, and billboard advertisement with one goal: *convince us to spend our hard earned money on products that are unconditionally guaranteed to keep pace with the young, the beautiful, and the desirable.*

Underlying YAAVIST is results: put *successful* looking, *visually young and attractive* people together with *thin bodies* and you have *sex* and plenty of it. (See: Reality TV, and the billion dollar-a-year porn industry.)

Morally "Fuzzy"

Then, there's morality. A permissive society like Pop Culture USA is subject to a variety of interpretations including the latest expression for propaganda, **pop semantics**—"whatever I say or appear to be in public is true, regardless" (whether or not it is actually true). Interestingly, the guru of popular semantics is, of course, former President Bill Clinton, known for "I didn't inhale" (marijuana)—or—"I did not have sex with that intern." After eight years of hearing "spin" from his morally ambivalent staff—"after all Bill and Monica are both adults—it is no wonder American citizens are a little "**morally fuzzy.**"

■ Incompetent Parenting—Far from Antisocial Parenting

Antisocial parenting aside, what should society expect from whiny, pampered kids raised by *incompetent* (yet caring) parents who lead them to believe society owes them something because they are so special (without accomplishing anything). Showing love and concern, with little or no skills for parenting, incompetent parenting is still far removed from the emotional and developmental devastation of hateful antisocial parenting. Antisocial kids hate everybody and everything in authority. The really sick ones worship at the "altar" of violent video games—not just playing them but becoming obsessed by them to the point of seeking to create personalized versions. They collect bizarre websites of deviant sexuality and are jazzed by violent, decadent, and depressing songs just like the Columbine "Rambo" killers Eric Harris (eighteen-years-of-age) and Dylan Klebold (seventeen-years-of-age).

Named for the "Rambo" character in the movie by the same name, Rambo stalked enemy with pop culture persona and pumping testosterone. Young kids and adolescents who kill—"Rambo" killers—seem to step out of video games with "do-rags," black high top boots, trench coats, and guns blazing, seething with **ethnocentrism**. Some prefer less of a grand entrance as they kill ex-girlfriends, peers, gays, or lesbians—anyone different—in vacant fields, bodies left behind for vermin and vultures. No person, especially so young, has this coming.

Blatant Hedonism

Reared in Pop Culture USA, nurtured by hedonistic values and sexual immorality, living by the creed, "it's ok to do it, as long as you don't get caught," young, adolescent killers are compulsive liars and compulsive cheaters. Right now, neuroscientists are showing they suffer from *irreversible neurological brain abnormalities*. They don't just *play* violent video games, they are *obsessed* with them. They get "jazzed" by violence in all its forms in a dizzying cocktail of chemistry surging from their own pleasure pathways of brain chemistry

Some pre-teens are so neurologically dysfunctional that they cannot separate lies from truth, fact from fiction. In general, regarding cognition (thinking and thoughts occurring in **internal dialogue**), how is *quality of thinking* conditioned? And, does quality of thinking influence behavior?

◼ Tolman: Making Sense Out of Mazes

Edward Chance Tolman spent most of his career at the University of California, Berkeley. Tolman coined the term *cognitive mapping* as a consequence of studying *behavior* in rats. Tolman's perspective—**purposive behaviorism**—brings cognitive theory into the midst of behaviorism. In his famous "cognitive mapping" study, one group of rats was placed in *various* "start" locations within the maze with food placed *in the same location* for each trial. The rats quickly learned the maze.

Another group of rats had food placed in *different locations* (with the same exact left and right turns as the other rats.) The rats with food in the same location performed much better than the group with food placed randomly in different locations. Tolman believed the rats had learned the *exact location* of the food due to experience and cognitive anticipation, rather than just a series of left and right turns. In other words, the group developed an internal, *goal-directed cognitive map* for the location of the food. The other group performed less effectively because they lacked an internal cognitive "locator."

Just like rats, humans are *goal-directed* and they seek the *shortest path to reach goals*. Tolman contends this set of conditions is due to the development of powerful *cognitive maps of learning*. We find our cars on a crowded parking lot by noticing landmarks; we can visualize a double-decker strawberry shortcake sundae with whipped topping in stark visualization (to the point we salivate), and we can race over to the downtown courthouse in our hometown without looking for road sign "locators" due to cognitive "maps."

Thus, empirically demonstrated in rats running in mazes, the development of cognitive mapping is no longer speculative, even in humans. Deviant cognitive maps from antisocial parenting, coupled with neurological damaged brains, can be devastating to individuals targeted as victims.

◼ Rapacious Cognitive Maps

The *quality of thinking* influences behavior (and vise-versa as behavior influences thinking) in powerful ways and is instrumental in the development of happy, well-adjusted children versus the rapacious mindset of adolescent "Rambo" killers, female killers, and male serial rapists and murderers. Imagine the impoverished and twisted cognitive maps of adolescents *obsessed* with guns, pipe bombs, explosives, sexually deviant websites, violent video games, perverse song lyrics of doom, death, and destruction. What do we expect will happen?

Expecting psychopathic kids to be honest with anyone amounts to delusional thinking. They embrace *hidden emotional agendas*. Any reference to peers, such as co-conspirators or references to experiences, such as making pipe bombs, explosives, deviant websites, or music is sure to be met with complete deception due to the intense *emotional investment* made by the kids in these scurrilous activities.

Early in development, psychopaths master the art of manipulation and lying. They lie right to your face. They look straight into your eyes and never blink. They offer to society a demeanor that is extremely effective at deception. As a society, we had better start looking behind the smiling faces or *blunt affect* (lack of emotional expression) that typifies severe psychopathy.

"Rambo" killers often start with petty crimes—vandalism and theft—and finish with major ones in home and schoolplace violence just like Harris and Klebold. With neurological brain irregularities, it is not conceivable by modern neuroscience to undo years of *systematic abuse and neglect* in antisocial families where perverted cognitive maps have taken over as cognitive "focusers". Until they weed themselves out by committing violence and landing in juvenile detention, prison, or in shootouts with police, society is not safe.

On the other hand, a child surrounded by emotionally nourishing activities with attentive, supportive, and loving family members and friends (even with a touch of incompetent parenting on occasion) develop a far different set of cognitive maps. The behaviorist John B. Watson thought so as well with his famous view of rearing children:

> "Give me a dozen healthy infants, well-formed, and my own specific world to bring them up in and I'll guarantee to take any one at random and train him to become any type of specialist I might select—doctor, lawyer, artist, merchant, and yes, beggar-man and thief, regardless of his talents, penchants, tendencies, abilities, vocations, and race of ancestors." (Watson, 1966).

◼ Grim Connection—Violence & Pseudo-Sapien Brains

The picture is a grim one. Home violence. School violence. The face of violence lives in many locations. In Austin, Texas a popular, bright, and vivacious sixteen-year-old girl decides to break up with her jealous and possessive boyfriend. He pulls a knife and stabs her to death in a hall of Reagan High School.

Several years ago, two high school seniors living near Ft. Worth conspired to kill a female classmate because the boy's girlfriend was jealous. The female killer thought her boyfriend and the female victim had sex. Lured away from the safety of her home, the teenage victim was shot and her head was bashed in. She died in a vacant field. Before the secret was known, both killers were accepted into our country's most prestigious service academies. Now, careers and lives ruined, they sit in federal prison. Recently, the female killer asked permission to marry a fellow inmate.

"Rambo" Killers Target the Face

In 1979, long before the 1990s—the decade of accelerated schoolplace violence—a seventeen-year-old female entered an elementary school and shot eight children and a police officer with a rifle she received as a Christmas present. Two men lost their lives trying to shield the children. After the six-hour siege ended, she told authorities "I don't like Mondays."

In 1987, a twelve-year-old boy brought a pistol to school and killed the boy who tormented him. Then, he killed himself. Then, the 1990s arrived.

Violent Vignettes

In 1993 in Kentucky, a seventeen year-old male, using his father's pistol in the attack, shot his teacher in the head and later a janitor. He held his classmates hostage. He disliked his teacher's comments on his book report of Stephen King's novel *Rage,* about a similar scenario.

In 1995 three separate incidences of schoolplace violence occurred. The first occurred in California where a thirteen year-old male, distraught over having to wear a school uniform, stole a shotgun from a friend, returned to school, and shot the principal in the face. Then he committed suicide. In South Carolina, a sixteen-year old male shot a teacher in the face and then killed himself because he had been suspended from school for making "a vulgar hand gesture". In Tennessee, a seventeen-year-old male fatally shot a teacher in the face then killed another student and teacher. The reason? Academic problems and a traffic accident the day before.

In 1996, a thirteen-year-old honor student shot and killed two students and a teacher with a deer rifle he brought from home. One of the students killed had called him "a nerd." His parents were divorcing and he suffered from depression. He thought Oliver Stone's *Natural Born Killers* and Stephen King's *Rage* were "cool." He watched the Pearl Jam video "Jeremy"—about an outcast who commits suicide.

Four incidences of schoolplace violence occurred in 1997. In Alaska, a sixteen-year old student killed one student and a principal and wounded two other students with a shotgun. He was tired of being called pejorative names. The perpetrator's father was known as "Rambo of Alaska" due to his own violent behavior. In Mississippi, a sixteen-year-old male student stabbed his mother to death and then shot nine students at school, two of whom died, including his ex-girlfriend. He referred to himself as a "satanic assassin." The boy's idol was Adolf Hitler. Before the shooting, he tortured and killed his dog. In Kentucky, a fourteen-year-old boy shot and killed three students, wounding five others. He enjoyed the violent video games *Doom* and *Quake*. When wrestled to the ground following the shootings he cried, "Kill Me Now"! Finally, another fourteen-year-old male hid in the woods and shot and wounded two students. The reason? They picked on him.

In 1998 three violent schoolplace events occurred. A thirteen-year-old male and an eleven-year-old male fatally shot four students and a teacher, wounding ten others. All victims were female. They stole seven handguns and three rifles from relatives. In the stolen van, police found sleeping bags, a radio, and a stuffed animal. In Pennsylvania, a fourteen-year-old suicidal boy shot and killed a teacher and wounded two students and a teacher. In Oregon, a fifteen-year-old murdered both his parents, who were teachers. He drove to school and fatally shot two students and wounded twenty-three others. He was tired of being teased, angry with his parents, and angry at the school. Indicative of some school administrators and school boards' denial of student violence, his middle school yearbook named him "Most Likely to Start World War III." *How to Build a Pipe Bomb* was his topic for a speech class.

In 1999, two violent schoolplace events occurred. In Georgia, a high school student injured six students with a rifle. He was on anti-depressant medication following a breakup with his girlfriend and failing grades. Directions on making bombs and explosives were found in his room. Then, in Colorado there was Columbine, the incident that raised the ante for schoolplace violence.

■ The Columbine Massacre

A cursory sketch follows in this section regarding what is known about the perpetrators of Columbine. Exemplified by arrogance, strategizing, bold maneuvering, and the sheer number of victims of the assailants (13 dead, 23 injured, and countless victims emotionally scarred for life) the massacre at Columbine High School stands as a reminder of the impact Pop Culture USA has on neurologically damaged brains.

The teenage perpetrators were loners who were called names by their peers—"inbreeds," "dirtbags," and "faggots." They associated with a group of peer malcontents known by the cool pop culture moniker "trench coat mafia." Harris and Klebold were obsessed with sexually deviant websites. They did not merely play video games; rather they were *obsessed* to the extent one of the killers customized a segment for his own enjoyment.

A few days before the killings, the Marines rejected Harris due to his prescription of psychiatric medication. Harris created his own website for his tortured psyche, including directions on how to make a pipe bomb with the cryptic message "goodbye to all on April 20th"—the date of the Columbine massacre. Looking back in 20/20 hindsight, prescient "red flags" were littered everywhere (as they always are) from home to school to websites in virtually reality. Who's paying attention to our children?

Both boys had prior felony convictions for breaking into a van. A parent complained about the website and harassment against his son to the police who forwarded a memo to the school. *No action was taken.*

Due to an established policy contending media hype contributes to increased crimes, the *Chicago Sun* was the only newspaper in the country not to carry it on the front page. Due to the onslaught of media coverage, however, the story was recently listed as the third largest this century (Zinna, 1999).

A *killing team* of two perpetrators to reinforce each other, using both bombs and guns to extract the most damage, was a tactical departure from most instances of schoolplace violence. Both boys had studied carefully the layout of the school and knew exactly where the greatest concentration of students would be—cafeteria and library—at the 11:00 A.M. strike hour. Showing blatant disregard for life, they calmly talked and joked with each other as they stalked (sometime killing victims hiding under desks). They killed victims fleeing for their lives. And, just as quickly as it had begun, the rampage was over.

■ Schoolplace Offender Profile

In 1998, the FBI developed the *schoolplace offender profile.* Intended as a general measure of *violent risk potential,* profilers caution that schoolplace violence is evolving and perhaps escalating. The following list of fourteen characteristics represents the type of behavior characteristic of "Rambo" killers:

1. White male, 17 years of age or younger, lacks discipline
2. Fascination with firearms and/or explosives,
3. Cruelty to pets,
4. Believes mother (or other family member) disrespects them,
5. Seeks to defend narcissistic view of self,
6. A depressed suicidal ideation turned homicidal by a triggering event—failed romantic relationship, lack of support from family, rejection, or revenge,
7. History of expressed anger or acts of physical aggression at school,
8. May have been influenced by satanic or cult type belief system,
9. May listen to music lyrics that promote violence,
10. May appear sloppy or unkempt in class,
11. May feel isolated from others,
12. May have a history of mental health treatment,
13. May feel powerless; may commit acts of violence to assert power over others,
14. May have openly expressed a desire to kill others, and
15. Presents low-self esteem

Compiled from *After Columbine: A Schoolplace Prevention Manual* (1999, Zinna).

Today, *home schooling* looks better all the time when compared to suburban schools, doorways lined with metal detectors, in an attempt to keep our children from being massacred at school. But, who's going to stay home with the children when both parents work? The behavioral dynamics of so-called **latchkey children**—children left alone and unsupervised before and/or after school—is a glaring part of the problem. Some do just fine. But, there are always some who don't.

▪ Once upon a Time

It is not necessary to run a sociological or historical survey comparing the *zeitgeist* of 1950s–1960s to 1990s–2000s. The current generation's parents or grandparents are acquainted with the time frame. Once upon a time, students respected teachers and coaches. Teachers had control of the classroom. In many American families, moms stayed home and raised the kids; dads worked—great arrangement. *Values, morals, and structure were central to schoolplace milieu* where students stood to the Pledge of Allegiance followed by a morning prayer in the classroom. Parents did not flock to the school to demand this tradition be stopped. Once upon a time, atheists filed no lawsuits to stop any procedures in the classroom.

Few students were disruptive, certainly not by today's standards. If they were, the boys (and some girls) got "licks" by a wooden paddle for inappropriate behavior. In fact, if boys didn't get a few paddles from the true "board" of education, classmates considered him too much of a "momma's boy", but his behavior was not hateful or rapacious. Now, parents are ready to sue if anyone paddles their little darlings. With little if any meaningful discipline at school or home, why are we shocked when kids take matters into their own hands?

Harking back to the past, in the 1960s, family budgets and economics made sense. A new Mustang automobile cost approximately $2,500 or less. A new four-bedroom home with approximately 1800 square feet cost under $20,000 (less than $10.00 a square foot to build). Once upon a time, the numbers worked.

Families had "dinner time" to socialize and share the activities of the day. (A few risk-takers ventured away from the table into the living room to watch TV with their food on the solitary "TV trays.")

At first, at least, most family members chose the comforting mix of food and conversation. Who has time to sit down at a meal today with family members? Tabulating how much our children spend a month on gas to-and-from fast food restaurants and the cost of the food might bring on a migraine.

Today, **cynicism** is rampant in schools. Teachers are laughed at and openly ridiculed. "Sue me," students say. Parents seem to be in a quandary of what to do. Parents of normal kids are in denial of the severity of pseudo-sapiens—kids with wrecked neurological systems—clandestinely stalking them. Incompetent parents in parent-teacher conferences act shocked that their kids act out in class even though they know their children have emotional issues. Constant fighting, insufficient money, and/or impending divorce hit the kids right between the eyes every morning. Who will they live with? What's going to happen? Will they ever see their friends again? Antisocial parents, who have severely emotionally scarred their children by abuse, emotional neglect, and hateful parenting never show up for conferencing. The kids may or may not attend school regularly.

In every way, teachers represent the "Rodney Dangerfield" of education—*they get no respect*. Students bully teachers and fellow students who are considered "nerds." Students control the classroom. Decency, morals and ethics went away a long time ago. Some political historians contend the meltdown occurred as a "trickle down effect" from the top leadership of our country beginning in the late 1970s when Nixon told his country, "I am not a thief!" Trickle down continued years later with Clinton's finger wagging to a national audience—"I did not have sex with that intern." Yes, Nixon was a liar and so was Clinton. Then, some observers say we must expect "minor" dishonesties from politicians. Who's left to blame for moral ineptitude? Are **litigious** atheists really responsible for the moral decay in our homes and schools?

Recently, an elementary school kid brought a gun to school. He showed it off; miraculously, the gun didn't discharge. The story goes that the kid's father is long on money and the school is short on memory. School officials did nothing over the protests of his classmates' parents. As a society, we already know you can get away with murder if you have money and influence.

Tongue-in-cheek, some nutritionists say the emotional problems students have in school is due to all the fat they eat in school cafeterias, especially fried foods and pizza. Many students become obese before the sixth grade. It is projected that one in three kids will be diabetic by age ten; one in two will be diabetic in black and Hispanic children. True, the high content of fat in fried foods clogs arteries and sensibilities—what about the brain?

Then there's the argument that all the toxins students breathe from carpet fibers and poor circulation of air found in even the most modern school buildings cause students to "act out." Has the alarming record number of allergies in children to do with airtight classrooms and carpeting? Voluminous studies have shown that fluorescent lighting causes hyperactivity in some children and inattentiveness in others. Still classrooms are lighted with fluorescent lights. It's cheaper.

Sadly, as statistics show, the 13-to-18-year-old-age group—middle school and high school aged kids—is the age group littered with perpetrators of schoolplace violence. Academically, critics of public education contend that *high school is a mind-numbing experience*. Critics maintain if you take time to ask kids whether or not high school prepared them for college, the first thing they do is laugh, and the second thing they do is ask "are you kidding?" No one seems to mind.

Perhaps years ago, some high schools believed their mission was to be a "prep" school—preparing students for college—a logical mission statement. Few argue today that high school has been reduced to "the last gasp" for extra-curricular activities, sports, and socializing, before the "seriousness" of college.

Critics further maintain that *high school is mostly about academic boredom*. Everybody knows only nerds study. "No pass, no play" has become a national joke no one takes seriously. Social historians are at a loss to explain the tectonic shift away for the "prep" school mission to idyllic Hormone High.

Today, in the home, both parents usually work. Budgets are always tight, as most families live pay-check-to-pay-check, hand to mouth. Credit cards are bloated due to high interest rates and irresponsible spending. Today, a new Mustang costs $40,000 dollars or more and a new four-bedroom 1,800 square-foot home costs approximately $180,000 (or $100 a square foot to build.) While salaries have gone up, many citizens' "standard of living" reflects the 1970s standard. Who has time for parenting? With parents working, bills to pay, and kids to raise, stress is over-the-top. *Emotional burnout is a silent epidemic in North America.*

Using examples from Eriksonian stage theory (from Chapter Four), we present compelling arguments in the development of adolescent killers primarily across three stages—Stage One: *Trust versus Mistrust;* Stage Four *Industry versus Inferiority;* and Stage Five *Identity versus Role Confusion,* where we highlight damaging effects of horrific parenting. Serial killers emerge in Stage Six, where the *emotional crisis of intimacy versus isolation* tips the scales toward sexualized violence.

■ Infancy: Trust versus Mistrust

Trust & Competent Parenting

No one expects to get an answer back from a one-year-old infant when asked, "Do you trust me?" But, the answer—in body language—is there nonetheless. When infants are attended to and nurtured by loving parents, when they are put on a predictable schedule of sleep and feeding, they are held, rocked, loved, touched, talked to and played with, when parents devote quality time away from the busy adult world, the result is predictable: children feel safe, secure, loved, and they trusts caregivers. They feel valued. Even mothers who retain their jobs (as observed in various *Mommy Tracks* available with many employers), they choose to breast feed their infants for at least three or four months to insure her infant's immune system gets nature's boost. A supportive husband, competent sitters, and attentive grandparents give her needed breaks.

Effective parenting is exhausting as well as exhilarating. The couple and infant *feel like family.*

Infancy Mistrust

Contrast the neurologically tweaked development of the infant during his/her first year of life. Antisocial, hateful parenting, conveying in body language alone a far different message to her child. First, Mom may have used drugs during pregnancy—legal as well as illegal. If she smoked cigarettes on a regular basis, the infant is born addicted to nicotine; if she drank alcohol on a consistent basis, the infant is an alcoholic addicted to ethanol. We have read newspaper accounts and TV documentaries of the horror of "crack babies." *Addicted mothers give birth to addicted infants.* Addicted infants cry and cry for weeks as they battle addiction and the awful withdrawal, further alienating insecure mothers. Addicted infants don't thrive well and they don't appear to feel secure and happy. They don't feel and look like they trust "caregivers."

Antisocial "father" figures may have walked (or more descriptively "run away") from responsibility, as psychopaths are prone to do, leaving the mother alone, tense, and afraid. She communicates negative feelings to her unborn infant. Perhaps her family disowned her or made it clear "you made your bed, now sleep in it." If the "father" remained in the picture he may be immature, ambivalent, and/or battling some kind of addiction himself.

In contrast to the nurturing couple, incompetent couples do *not feel like family.* They may feel trapped, cheated, or unlucky. Why did this have to happen to us? Immature and incompetent male "fathers" shun their pregnant girlfriends so they can keep partying with their equally immature and incompetent "friends." Some have poisoned their pregnant girlfriends to "get rid of the problem."

New mothers may be uncomfortable with breastfeeding, so bottle-feeding will have to do. Finding a formula that agrees with her child is often a "hit and miss" proposition. She may not be sure what to do when her baby cries. Often, supportive grandparenting is absent and she cannot afford competent sitters. Within months, very young mothers who have little or no support systems are tense, nervous, and exhausted. Mothers who raise their child alone often have limited funds and may have limited understanding of effective parenting skills. Routinely propping a bottle under a folded diaper to feed her infant lying flat on his/her back while the exhausted mom tries to take a short nap is an exercise in futility. The slightest movement of the infant's head in the wrong direction will displace the nipple from mouth to ear, if the nipple has not already collapsed. Crying acts like a demonic "alarm clock" to the stressed-out mother.

■ Stage Four—Formal Schooling

Traditionally, *successful transition from the home milieu to the school milieu* is considered a benchmark accomplishment of normalcy in our society. It is considered dysfunctional when students make a poor transition, become truant and/or oppositional defiant. Something is missing. In stage Four, *Industry versus Inferiority* (six-years-old to twelve-years of age), normal children come to expect *predictability* from teachers and *formal schooling* as well as from parents. Social and academic success comes in stages or rather grade levels, as normal kids manage tasks related to the level of learning expectations. Dysfunctional children *never like school;* mostly, they are academically weak and socially aloof, seldom achieving more than "average."

Elementary and middle school teachers see the "red flags" of dysfunctional parenting as troubled children act differently than normal kids. (Home schooling has been shown to be an effective alternative to public or private education. Recently, the author was asked to speak at a commencement exercise of home-schooled students. Talented children performed vocally and on musical instruments while devoted parents watched gleefully the highlights of the evening. Families gathered together on stage to celebrate promotion to the next grade level. *There is no question that home schooling provides an effective alternative to the "cookie-cutter" factory of public school education.*

◼ Stage Five: Twelfth Year through Eighteen Year—The Rise of "Rambo" Killers

In this stage, even with limited perspective and maturity, normal children come to see themselves as *unique individuals* with "upsides and downsides". They understand the "pecking order" of high school with its predictable clicks and stereotypes. Some find it amusing as involved parents have given good advice: *high school is not the real world.* Other kids find the pecking order of high school unfair, irritating, or humorous, but only the kid with *features* of psychopathic personality is at the extreme—he either loves it (too much) it or hates it (too much).

Mild Psychopathy—Not an Oxymoron

In fact, some of the most popular high school students have *features* of psychopathy. This does not mean they are going out in the world to be serial killers. It does mean they might be very successful in business, especially sales. *Psychopathic personality stretches across a wide continuum of mild, moderate, and severe features.* Sexual psychopaths (serial killers) are at the most extreme end of the psychopathy continuum. The "mild" and "moderate"—the garden variety psychopaths are covered in more detail in Chapter Eight.

Besides being physically attractive, individuals with mild psychopathic features display egocentricity (self-centeredness), narcissism, extraversion with a "gift of gab," superficial charm, emotional shallowness (which ironically guards against becoming discouraged by other's comments), and a self-styled fabrication of reality to suit them. Other less attractive and more introverted students (who are less popular in high school) often "blossom" as *late bloomers* in college. Immaturity and lack of perspective aside, many of the "red flags" of psychopathy are clearly visible by high school. Some students with mild features of psychopathy simply grow out of it as they mature and embrace the higher expectations of the college experience. Those not willing to adapt, adjust, or modify their "high school" mindset to the rigors of higher education are indicative of personality *rigidity* characterized by *faulty coping skills,* psychopathic traits.

Dropping out of high school has many causes but severe psychopathy cannot be ignored.

Along with ego integration, normal kids at this age start to trust their own "gut" feelings. They see a completely different world than the budding psychopath. With parental encouragement, they become connected or involved in some aspect of school or community that enriches and expands personality. They genuinely want to help others.

The loner psychopath may feel completely depersonalized (Erikson refers to it as *role confusion*). The "Rambo" killer-to-be feels detached, isolated, frustrated, and angry. He may have already displayed antisocial behavior by having to report to a probation officer, beating up a string of dysfunctional girlfriends, committing random acts of vandalism, being expelled from school, and/or by setting fires. He's one "triggering" event away from committing his first act of "Rambo" violence.

■ Females Who Kill

Female Serial Killers

Exposed to hateful and abusive antisocial parenting, boys and young adult males display violent behavior with pronounced oppositional defiance and behavioral deviance. In contrast, adolescent and young adult females typically "turn on themselves" and become sexually promiscuous, drug-addicted, passive or dependent with **borderline** or **histrionic** personality features. As noted earlier with the male variety, *Personality Disorder NOS (PD NOS)* is usually the most accurate clinical definition due to the presence of multiple personality disorders, exacerbated by poly-addiction. While female serial killers experience similar dysfunctional childhoods and abusive backgrounds, they show a pattern of not "acting out" aggressively as the male variety—rage is directed inward as *self-hatred*. Female killers tend to be spree killers, "heat of passion" killers, or retaliation killers. They often become chronically depressed and fall into addiction.

In 2003, as an example of "heat of passion" rage, a thirty-something female dentist repeatedly ran over her husband in her Mercedes-Benz in front of the hotel where he and his young girlfriend met for weekly sexual liaisons. Convicted of murder and given a 20-year prison sentence, she testified, "I didn't mean to run over him three times, I was aiming at his car." (Maybe she should have studied to be an ophthalmologist.)

In the 1990's Long Island "Lolita," Amy Fisher attempted to murder her seedy boyfriend's wife by shooting her in the face when she answered the door. In the 1980's Lorena Bobbitt severed her husband's penis while he slept. She said he was abusive. Following divorce, over a year later, an assault charge was filed against Lorena Bobbitt by a boyfriend. Given new life with an enhanced penis, John Wayne Bobbitt turned to *Pop Culture USA* and has become a star of porn movies.

Male serial killers kill strangers, while females kill people they know—husbands, nursing home residents, hospital patients, coworkers, kids in the neighborhood, or their own children.

Motives, Methods, Typology, and Profiles

Reviewing the literature, researchers agree that female serial killers are rare. According to one source, only 8% of all serial killers in America are female; however, the same 8% accounts for 76% of all female serial killers worldwide. Since 1970, a 57% increase in the number of male serial killers occurred, while in the same time period, the number of female serial killers increased by 138%! Yet, in **Mindhunter,** former FBI profiler John Douglas states, "The fact remains women do not kill *in the same way* or in anywhere remotely near the numbers men do."

What motivates female serial killers? Known for "maternal instincts" and nurturing, what happens in their minds to produce murdering predators? How does her MO differ from male serial killers? Does she display signature? What characterized her *modus vivendi?*

Interviews with female serial killers (Alarid, Marquart, Burton, and Cullen, 1996) uncovered the disturbing statistic that 86% of all female serial killers work in tandem with either a male or female *accomplice* (known as the **secondary follower role**). This fact accounts for a much different dynamic from the killer who acts alone.

The average amount of time before a female serial killer is apprehended is *eight years,* while men are caught in approximately half that time.

Kelleher & Kelleher (1998) describe the female serial killer as *successful, careful, precise, methodical, and quiet.* The favored *methods* and *motivation* of the female serial killer were first consistently identified by Hickey (2002). (Some killers used more than one method and displayed more than a single motive, so the percentages will be over 100%.)

Method Used:

Poison	80%
Shooting	20%
Bludgeoning	16%
Suffocation	16%
Stabbing	16%
Drowning	5%

Motive:

Money	74%
Control	13%
Enjoyment	11%
Sex	10%
Drugs	24%

Typology

As previously noted, scant research into the psychological or neurochemical aspects of female serial killers exists. According to Kelleher & Kelleher, the *organized/disorganized* typology of male serial killer is noticeably absent from female serial killer typology. Consequently, the researchers have developed a deductive nine-point categorization based on assessment of the two typologies of female serial killers—(1) females who act alone, and (2) females who acts in partnership with another (or others).

1. Females *acting alone* include:
   Black Widow
   Angel of Death
   Sexual Predator
   Revenger
   Profit/Crime

2. Females acting in partnership include:
   Team killers
   Insane killer (question of sanity)

3. Unexplained Killers

4. Unresolved Killers

Making an Argument

According to criminal profiling student Rae Ellen Wooten, PA, the Kelleher typology places three types of female serial killers—the "Question of Sanity" (Insane Killer), the "Unexplained" Killer, and the "Unsolved" Killer into *acting in partnership* typology. This appears to defeat the purpose of the typology, which is better suited for "acting alone/disorganized" category due to the *psychological aspects* manifested in the profiled cases. None of the three categories—Insane Killer, Unexplained Killer, and Unresolved Killer—include a partner. Hence, why "acting in partnership" typology?

Furthermore, the "unsolved" category simply does not supply enough information to attribute the crimes examined to a female killer at all, and for all practical purposes, should be omitted. Furthermore, the *acting alone* category (as defined by Kelleher & Kelleher) clearly represents the *organized* type of killer (as observed in the male variety). Therefore, it seems logical to modify the typologies as follows:

1. Acting alone (organized),
2. Acting alone (disorganized), and
3. Acting in partnership.

Acting Alone—Female Organized Serial Killer

This typology includes killers who are more mature, careful, deliberate, socially adept, and highly organized. These women usually attack victims in their home or place of work. Favored specific weapons include poison, lethal injection, or suffocation.

PREDATOR PROFILE (7-1)

The Dirty Dozen—11 Sketches of Females Who Kill & The Manson Family (7-2)

The "Black Widow"

"Black Widows" usually begin their career after age twenty-five. They progress to a cycle of systematically killing spouses, partners, family members, or anyone with whom they have developed a personal relationship. The typical cycle is six to eight victims over a period of ten to fifteen years. Poison is the preferred weapon or other lethal substances intended to mimic medication. The salient motive is greed, where the widow benefits from an inheritance or life insurance policy.

1. Margie Barfield, Dianna Lumbrera

A fifty-three-year old grandmother, Margie Velma Barfield (with crimes committed from 1969 to 1978) *killed seven husbands, fiancés, and her own mother* in North Carolina. She burned some victims to death while they slept, making it appear as though they were smoking in bed. She arranged prescription drug overdoses for some of the victims. She used arsenic to mimic gastroenteritis in others. She was executed by lethal injection in 1984, the first woman to be executed in the United States since 1976.

Dianna Lumbrera systematically *suffocated six of her own children* in Fort Worth, Texas from 1977 to 1990. The MO consisted of rushing each child (who was already dead) to the hospital and blaming the medical staff for not resuscitating the child. Initially, *Sudden Infant Death Syndrome,* or "crib-death" was suspected. Eventually, hospital officials became suspicious. She was tried, convicted, and sentenced to three life terms.

The "Angel of Death"

The "Angel of Death" begins her career around age twenty-one. She works in a localized medical setting—hospitals, nursing homes, or extended-care facilities—where death is a regular occurrence, along with life-sustaining, or life-terminating medications. In her camouflaged role of caregiver, murder can be easily disguised. The offender *enjoys the power of "playing God"* by selecting "who will live and who will die." The typical cycle is eight victims over a one to two year period. Angels of Death tend to brag about their crimes often bringing about their capture. The offender who moves from one facility to another may kill many more victims before being discovered.

2. Genene Jones

Genene Jones was a twenty-seven year old licensed vocational nurse (LVN) who specialized in the terminal care of pediatric patients. Jones was a highly mobile killer. She began her career in large metropolitan hospitals in San Antonio before migrating to other hospitals. She may have been responsible for as many as forty-six deaths from 1978 to 1982. Jones' MO consisted of injecting either the heart medication Digoxin® or the respiratory paralytic Pavulon® into infants. Then, she "discovered" the patient's distress. She enjoyed the attention she received from grateful co-workers and parents for her skill at resuscitating infants. After the CDC investigated her, she relocated to a physician's office in Kerrville. She went to trial in 1984 after the last patient she injected died en route to the hospital. The child had been brought to the clinic for routine immunizations. Jones' method included having the parent leave the room during the immunization stating that the child would be less inclined to cry. She injected the child with a lethal injection. Amazingly, her employment and medical records at several Texas institutions were illegally shredded to prevent further investigation and potential lawsuits.

Sexual Predator

Female sexual predators are so rare as to be an anomaly. Researchers are involved in extensive worldwide research to locate other offenders that fit this typography. Sexual predator Aileen Wournos may be the prototype of all future female sexual predators.

3. Aileen Wournos

Aileen Wournos, a 33-year-old prostitute living in Florida, killed seven men who solicited sex. (She was accused of two more murders, but the cases were never proven.) At some point in each sexual encounter, she perceived the sexual encounter to become abusive. As a remedy, she shot each victim repeatedly with a .22 caliber handgun, robbed him, and hid the body in the woods, along Florida's I-95 corridor. Her victims included men from all walks of life: a known rapist, two retired or reserve police officers, one missionary, two truck drivers, and deliverymen. She was apprehended by a careless paper trail she left from pawning items she collected during the robberies. At her trial in 1992, she claimed self-defense due to a childhood of physical and sexual abuse. Interestingly, her lesbian lover provided testimony against her disproving her claim of self-defense. She was sentenced to the electric chair.

A movie starring actresses Charlize Theron as Wournos, and Christina Ricci as her lesbian lover, will be released in the summer of 2003. The title of the movie is "Monster."

Revenge Killer

The common revenge killing is a *crime of passion*. However, the female revenge serial killer is very rare. What makes the revenge serial killer unique is the deep, pathological anger that drives the killer. There is little or no cooling-off period, implying an obsessive attachment to single-minded revenge. The revenge killer usually begins at about age twenty-two. Victims may include family members and/or symbols of an organization that the killer has deemed offensive, such as an abortion clinic. The usual pattern is three to four victims over a period of less than two years, although some killers may operate for up to five years. Although the revenge killer is usually capable of exerting enough control to conceal the crime, they are shown to be careless and demonstrate a lack of planning. Interestingly, they show great remorse when captured.

4. Martha Wise

Martha Wise, known as "the Borgia of America," was a 39 year-old widow who fell in love with a younger man to whom her family was opposed. One by one, she poisoned three of her family members before other relatives became suspicious and reported her to authorities. She confessed to the murders, several attempted murders, and to the arson of the church, which had been reluctant to permit her marriage ceremony. Her defense at trial was "the devil made me do it." She was sentenced to life imprisonment.

Profit/Crime Killer

Female serial killers motivated by profit or crime are also extremely rare. Some are thought to be organized contract killers for hire. Some have set up localized scam operations to rob victims. *They are considered to be the most intelligent, resourceful, and careful of all female serial killers.* Their careers begin at about age twenty-five or thirty and may last for ten years. They kill from ten to twenty-five victims before they are apprehended. This type of killer uses a variety of methods, and is dispassionate about the murders that she commits. *There are significantly more female killers of this genre worldwide than in the United States.*

5. Madame Popova, Anna Marie Hahn

Madame Popova perpetrated a murder-for-hire service in Russia specializing in killing cruel husbands for a fee. She is credited with achieving over 300 victims by means of poison, weapons, her own hands, or a hired assassin. She was apprehended when Russian police were informed by a remorseful widow; Madame Popova was executed by a firing squad for murders committed over an extended period from 1879–1909.

Anna Marie Hahn, twenty-six year old immigrant from Germany, worked in the Cincinnati area as a live-in caretaker for elderly men. Over a period of about five years, she bilked five victims out of their assets. She was also an expert in the utilization of poisons. She used different poisons to kill each victim. Her downfall came at the hands of suspicious bank examiners. Even though she utilized a mercy killing defense, she became the first woman in the history of Ohio to die in the electric chair in 1938.

Acting Alone—Disorganized Female Serial Killer

Severe *psychotic disorders* such as schizophrenia, and *substance abuse* disorders characterize this type of female killer. Extremely rare, prudent skepticism should be observed in labeling these murderers "disorganized". "Women come from the same backgrounds as males in the disorganized typology. Girls are even more subject to abuse and molestation than boys."

Question of Sanity—Insane Killers

This type of female killer thought to be insane is rare. While "Angel of Death" predators, who offer the psychological defense of **Munchausen Syndrome by Proxy,** may be the most successful in implementing the insanity defense, most killers, with question of sanity, are still convicted of first-degree murder.

6. Bobbie Sue Terrell, Andrea Yates

Bobbie Sue Terrell, a twenty-nine-year-old diagnosed schizophrenic, worked the nightshift as an employee of a nursing home. She used injections of insulin on each of twelve victims in St. Petersburg, Florida. After the murders, she mutilated herself, called police, and alleged an attack by a serial killer. She was arrested when police discovered her psychiatric background. She was judged insane and sentenced to sixty-five years in a clinical forensic prison.

On June 20th, 2001, Andrea Yates, a 37-year-old "post-op" nurse, murdered her five children by drowning them one by one. She had a long history of psychotic episodes, a diagnosis of schizophrenia, and recently had been diagnosed with *postpartum depression* after the births of her fourth and fifth children.

Yates' mother remarked that her daughter had always seemed isolated as a teenager. Her father was a teacher and a perfectionist. Yates' was consistently an academic over-achiever. She made great efforts to please her father. After the birth of her first child, she began having homicidal visions where knives and stabbings were prominently featured. On several occasions, she attempted suicide. She frequently had auditory hallucinations. Her family history includes two siblings with depression and another sibling diagnosed as bipolar. Despite a strong insanity defense, on March 13, 2002, a Houston jury took just 40 minutes to find her guilty of the deliberate murder of three of her five children. She was sentenced to life in prison.

Unexplained Motive—Neighborhood Killers

Neither the female serial killer, nor the authorities are able to discern a motive for these murders. In many instances, drug abuse may be the "trigger."

7. Christine Fallin, Audrey Hilley

Christine Fallin, a 17 year-old babysitter from Perry, Florida, murdered at least five neighborhood children by suffocation. She stated she heard voices telling her to commit the murders and prevent others from hearing the victims' scream. She was sentenced to life imprisonment for her crimes that occurred from 1980 to 1983. She will be eligible for parole in 2007.

Audrey Hilley, a 42 year-old housewife from Alabama used arsenic to poison several neighborhood children and family members. Three victims died, including some of her family, and several more became seriously ill. She claimed to suffer from bouts of "alternative consciousness" where she became her twin sister. She was judged insane. In prison she became a model inmate. After her release, she repeated her macabre behavior earning a life sentence.

Acting in Partnership—Female Serial Killers

Characteristics of this typology of female killers acting in partnership include killers who are younger, aggressive, vicious attackers, and sometimes disorganized, displaying evidence of a lack of careful planning. Victims are attacked in diverse locations. Torture is often involved before guns and/or knives are used to kill victim. In most instances, the female killer seems to be a follower rather than a leader, a dependent personality type, rather than the instigator.

Team Killer

The team killer type represents *one-third of all female serial killers,* and is subdivided into three subtypes of teams. Each category has an average murder count of nine to fifteen victims. A wide variety of weapons are used including guns and knives.

The three-team categories are (1) male-female, (2) female-female, and (3) family. Male-female teams are the most common and the most sexualized. The female member is usually about twenty years of age. She will have a short career of one to two years as a team killer.

8. Bonnie Parker & Clyde Barrow, Caril Ann Fugate & Charles Starkweather, Debra Brown & Alton Coleman

Bonnie Parker (16-years-of-age) and Clyde Barrow (21-years-of-age) began a crime spree in Dallas, Texas that extended into six states—Oklahoma, Kansas, Missouri, Iowa, Arkansas, and Louisiana. Eventually, they formed a gang, stealing cars, robbing banks and grocery stores. Of the sixteen people they shot and killed, thirteen were police officers. "Bonnie and Clyde" were team killers between 1930–1934. Reportedly, Bonnie enjoyed putting a few extra bullets into the corpses of police officers. A movie of the team's exploits was made by actor/director Warren Beatty.

In 1958, Caril Ann Fugate (age 14) and Charles Starkweather (age 19), originally from Lincoln, Nebraska, embarked on a one-month crime spree in Nebraska and Wyoming. They shot and killed eleven people including Caril's family. They ate and had sex for three days in the same house with the dead bodies of her family. Charles committed rape with at least one female victim before shooting her. Caril reportedly mutilated the genitals of this same victim in a jealous rage. They were captured in a high-speed car chase. Charles was sentenced to die by electrocution in 1959. Caril was incarcerated for 20 years. Two Hollywood movies—*Badlands,* and *Natural Born Killers,* were based on the team killers exploits.

In 1984, Debra Brown (age 21) and Alton Coleman (28 year-old, ex-con), African-American, common law couple from Chicago targeted African-American victims in a seven-week crime spree. The killings took place in Illinois, Indiana, Michigan, and Ohio. Ranging in age from seven to forty-one, eight of the victims were brutally raped and murdered. Alton had a history of being an aggressive "pansexual." The couple made the FBI's most wanted list. They each received multiple death sentences in three states.

Female Killer Teams

Female team killers are typically 25 years-of-age. They kill for two to four years until apprehended.

9. Gwendolyn Graham & Catherine May Wood

In 1987, Gwendolyn Graham (age 24) and Catherine May Wood (age 25), a lesbian couple, achieved sexual thrills in killing five elderly female patients at a nursing home where they were employed. Their MO was to suffocate the victim. Their signature consisted of making love immediately afterwards, thereby enhancing the intensity and thrill of sex. Wood was the submissive one, while Graham was the dominant, sexually exploitative partner. When Graham left her lover to take a job out of state, Wood confessed to the crimes. Graham received life imprisonment while Wood was incarcerated for twenty years.

Unsolved Killers—UNSUB (Unidentified Subject)

10. UNSUB "The Butcher of Kingsbury Run",
UNSUB Angel of Death "muscle relaxant" murder

From 1935–1938, twelve men were murdered by castration and decapitation along a stretch of railroad between Cleveland and Pittsburgh. The UNSUB became known as "The Butcher of Kingsbury Run." Was the murderer a male or female serial killer or team killers? At the time, popular sentiment speculated the decapitation murders were the work of just one woman.

In 1975, five murders were accomplished by injection of a muscle relaxant. The drug was somehow administered by intravenous tube, even when the patients were under close observation by hospital officials. The FBI and CDC were also involved in the investigation. It was believed that a technologically savvy "Angel of Death" was operating in the hospital, but no suspects were ever identified.

Family Team of Killers—Female Serial Killers

Female killers are about 20 years of age when family team of killers begin. The family teams last about a year before being apprehended. Prior to *Predator Profile (7-2),* which presents Charles Manson and his teenage "family", the most famous of Family Killer Teams, the McCreary team, follows.

11. McCrary Family Killers

In 1971–1972, the McCrary Family consisting of Carolyn and Sherman McCrary, their son Daniel, their daughter and son-in-law, Ginger and Ray Taylor, were responsible for the rape and shootings of twenty-two victims, mostly young female employees of stores robbed from Florida to California. They repeatedly raped the victims in the car, shot them, and threw the bodies out the window of the speeding car.

They were caught after a police shoot-out in Santa Barbara, California. The FBI linked them to twelve additional unsolved homicides, although they were only convicted of ten murders.

Female Killers Compiled By:

Rae Ellen Wooten, PA, criminal profiling student

PREDATOR PROFILE (7-2)

Charles Manson
"The Manson Family"

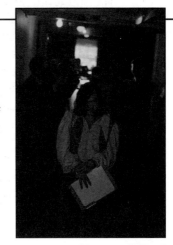

©Bettman/CORBIS

The Manson "family" committed horrific crimes that shocked the nation in 1968–1969. The crimes were referred to as "crimes of the century." The first five murders comprised what investigators called "The Tate Murders." Actress Sharon Tate, wife of movie producer Roman Polanski (*Chinatown, The Pianist*), was eight months pregnant at the time of the murders. Tate and Hollywood hair stylist Jay Sebring were found inside the sprawling LA mansion with a rope tied around their necks and slung around a ceiling rafter. She died from sixteen stab wounds to the chest and back. Sebring died from multiple stab wounds and one gunshot wound. Coffee heiress Abigil Folger and boyfriend Voytek Frykowski were found dead on the back lawn. Frykowski died from multiple stab wounds, two gunshot wounds, and head trauma from being severely beaten. Folger was stabbed a total of twenty-eight times. Steven Parent, the last victim, was found shot and stabbed to death in his car.

The next night, two more murders occurred and later were identified as the "LaBianca Murders." Grocery store magnate Leo LaBianca and his wife Rosemary were found stabbed to death in their home. He had been stabbed multiple times. The word "war" was cut into his flesh, a knife and fork protruded from his body. Rosemary had been stabbed forty-one times. Lamp cords were tied around the necks of both bodies. In the house on the three walls "Death To Pigs," "Rise," and Healther Skelter (misspelled) were found written in the victim's blood.

At the center of both murders revolved a bizarre looking thirty-four year-old ex-convict, Charles Manson who led the Manson "family"—comprised of teenagers. The principal members were Susan Atkins, Patricia Krenwinkel, Leslie Van Houten, Mary Brunner, Linda Kesabian, Lynette "Squeaky" Fromme, and Charles "Tex" Watson, a prep school football star. Manson directed, but never participated, in any of the Tate-LaBianca murders. The 1970 trial in LA resulted in guilty verdicts and the death penalty for all members. Later, the death sentences were automatically commuted to life sentences due to the Supreme Court ruling the death penalty unconstitutional.

The "family" may have totaled 50 to 100 members at one time. Manson was the illegitimate son of a sixteen-year-old girl addicted to alcohol and drugs. He never knew his father; his only male role model was an uncle, a rough "mountain man" who was deeply prejudiced. After several stints in prison, Manson lived with his strictly religious aunt in West Virginia. He was a bright child with an IQ of 109 but, at first, emotionally struggled with illegitimacy, his small physical size, and lack of parental love. Though he had little formal schooling, he was articulate, charming, and bright. He was a textbook psychopath.

He "acted out" by stealing and was sent to reform school at age nine. At age thirteen, he and another boy committed two armed robberies. As a teenager, he was "criminally sophisticated" despite his age. He had spent so much time in jail; some authorities believed he felt "institutionalized" by his mid-twenties. In prison, he enjoyed walking in the yard and playing his guitar.

In the psychedelic drug culture of the 1960s, Manson learned about drugs—primarily LSD and amphetamines—and how he could use them to influence people. Many of his "family" were young women with troubled emotional pasts, rebelling against parents and society.

Manson loved music. For a time, he hung out with Dennis Wilson of the Beach Boys. He failed to impress Wilson and others with his music. To this day, he blames this failure for plunging him into the dark side of paranoia. The Tate-LaBianca murders followed. The Manson "family" carried out his plan of Helter Skelter—following a devastating race war. Manson believed his "family" could emerge and taking control of society.

Manson Family "hit list" emerged. The list included actor Richard Burton who was to be castrated. Actress Elizabeth Taylor would have her eyes cut out and the words "Helter Skelter" carved by a hot knife into her forehead. The plan called for a jar containing Taylor's eyes and Burton's penis to arrive in the mail at Eddie Fisher's home (Taylor's ex-husband). Frank Sinatra was to be skinned alive listening to his own music. They planned to use his skin to make women's purses. Finally, singer Tom Jones' throat would be slit, after being forced to have sex with "family" member Atkins.

◾ A Breed Apart

Death Row Romance—Women Who Love Serial Killers

Sexual predators are among the most dangerous human monsters alive. By rapacious behavior, they seek to cause pain and suffering on mostly female victims, who are often oblivious to the propensity of a human to commit such extreme sexualized violence. Who would dare love such shameless creatures lurking behind a human face?

Some women claim their romantic relationships with death row inmates (many of whom are serial killers) evolved out of protests to end the death penalty in the United States. However, this rationalization seems too antiseptic, considering the *passionate love letters* many inmates receive.

"Death row inmates are held like animals. They can only step outside twice a week for two hours, and can only take showers three times per week for five minutes; their cells are tiny," says Andrea Faust, an inmate's soon-to-be-wife.

Other women claim they feel empathy toward the inmates because of loss of contact with family and friends. Why would these women become romantically engaged (in their own minds) with violent rapists and killers they will never be allowed to physically touch? Also, conjugal visits are out of the question.

Jan Arriens, founder of an organization called *Lifelines,* believes "women who love criminals" have something to do with the *dysfunctional relationships* these women had with their fathers, former boyfriends, or ex-husbands. Arriens claims that many of the women suffered *some form of abuse* at the hands of a man; consequently, they relate *romantic infatuation or love to violence.* He also feels that change occurs over long periods of time and the inmates are reaching out for women to understand them. As they age, death row inmates physically change, but psychologically, they remain the same.

Women who love criminals will continue to write and visit death row inmates as long as they are permitted, whether out of sympathy or some misunderstood passion. The women and the romantic passion shown for death row inmates are almost as scary as the incarcerated human monster himself. But, matters of the heart—especially the bruised and abused heart—remain the least understood aspect of human behavior for psychologists as well as criminal profilers.

Compiled by: Sonia Todd, criminal profiling student

Aftermath

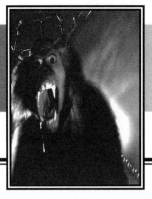

I. Word Scholar

Define the following words from *The Word Scholar Glossary*.

1. Pop culture USA _____

2. Pseudo-intellectual _____

3. Neurotheology _____

4. Consumerism _____

5. Pop semantics _____

6. Ethnocentricism _____

7. Cynicism _____

8. Hedonistic features _____

9. Borderline features _____

10. Secondary follower role _____

II. The Forensic Lab

Compose a one page report addressing: Speculate why females turn horrific parenting "inward" as self-hatred and why males turn horrific parenting "outward" against strangers as serial killers. In the alternative, why do females adopt the secondary follower role and as compliant co-offenders?

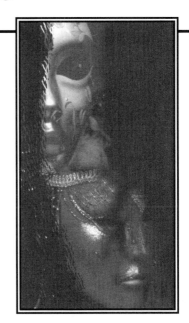

CHAPTER 8

The Mark of the Beast

❝*As it was, the skin emollient did it. She knew who had her then. The knowledge fell on her like every scalding awful thing on earth and she was screaming, screaming, under the futon, up and climbing, clawing at the wall, screaming until she was coughing something warm and salty in her mouth . . .***❞**

—*Silence of the Lambs*
Thomas Harris

"When he started killing women, he actually breathed life back into a couple of them, because they lost consciousness too quickly. He said, 'I wasn't going to let myself be robbed of the experience. I wanted to see in her eyes that she knew she was going to die, and that I was going to take her life . . .'"

—Janet Warren, Dept. of Behavorial Medicine and Psychiatry, University of Virginia (Discussing the confessions of a serial killer)

◼ Stay Close. Go Far.

At Weatherford College, a popular marketing slogan reads: "Stay Close. Go Far." The four-word slogan succinctly sums up the value of acquiring a quality education by staying close to home. Applying this to serial sexual psychopathy, if authorities "stay close" to criminal profiling, forensic evidence, and imaging from brain scanning technology, we "go far" in piecing together the puzzle of society's most elusive predators. Since safe neighborhoods no longer exist, parents who "stay close" to their children and keep them in view as much as possible will "go far" in preventing the need to profile a targeted offender. Stay Close. Go Far—aphoristically, true. With serial killers on the loose,

213

something's got to give. As a culture, we are heading into Huxley's "brave new world" of prevention and strategizing—new ways of making this planet safe for all of us, especially women and children. We subscribe to **prescient** thinking—*an ounce of prevention is worth a pound of cure*.

Interspersed with brief summations of preceding chapters regarding the puzzle of sexual psychopathy, we offer our analyses and comments. The danger of our beautiful children crossing the path of a serial killer comprises the *sum of all parental fear*. First, to what we know.

▪ Differentiation

Not all individuals with a psychopathic personality (or psychopathic features) have antisocial personality disorder. While they are not violent criminals or pedophiles, they may be highly successful "con men" or ruthless business executives, "psychopaths in suits". However, all sexual psychopaths (serial killers) are sexual predators with antisocial personality disorder, and lots more. "Milder" forms of psychopathy may be what Darwin meant by his term "survival of the fittest". Perhaps individuals, characterized by grandiosity of self and lack of empathy or care for others, may have an advantage in physically surviving as the most emotionally fit. Interesting conjecture.

Non-criminal psychopaths are glib—literally "slippery"—and possess an engaging personality. They are often magnets to women of all ages searching for an exciting relationship. *Feeling safe is the danger* of sustained interaction with "mild" or "moderate" psychopaths, as they are both disarming and flattering at first. For some individuals, *being around the most engaging ones is like an addiction*. They are a hard habit to break. Due to their pleasing persona, they catch victims off guard. Some psychopaths are overly theatrical in expression, while the sexual psychopath projects **flat affect** (emotionless expression), reflecting neurological damage. *Sexual psychopaths* will kill you. No conscience. No remorse. No problem. But, there's more.

Perversion of sexuality by deviant cognitive maps of thinking, largely due to obsessive-compulsive addiction to hardcore violent pornography, or in the alternative, repression of normal sexuality (due to a hateful, domineering mother) often results in a child obsessed with sex and sexual fantasies. Serial killer Ed Gein's mother forbade him from even looking at women, which had the opposite effect of creating an obsession for females, especially nude females. Gein's mother felt females were at the root of all sin. As soon as Gein had the house to himself he set out to discover "why." In sexual repression, by the teenage years, obsession may turn to *compulsion* and the desire to possess the object of the obsession. But there's more.

Kids who grow up to become serial killers start the developmental process in severely dysfunctional homes, highlighted by abuse and emotional dysfunction. In what we have termed antisocial parenting—loveless, hateful, and hurtful parenting characterized by physical abuse—children are "knocked around" hit on the head, shoved down stairs, slapped in the face, knocked up against walls, or generally "beat" upon. Most of these children experience further damage from sexual abuse. "Rewiring" the brain does not have to be the result of pure physical abuse alone; emotional abuse can result in irreversible neurological damage in ways we are beginning to understand. Head trauma is especially neurologically devastating, especially before two years of age, as observed in variations of the *shaken baby syndrome.*

The brain floats in cerebrospinal fluid with no specific gravity of its own. Hence, trauma to the head results in the brain's prefrontal lobes being forced violently against the bony cranium. This jarring effect, if violent enough, produces a neurological "ding" to the cortices, resulting in neurological trauma of the "cool-coded" variety. In Chapter One, the brain scans of Donta Page and Jeremy Skotz reflected "cool-coding" of trauma. How many incarcerated serial killers show similar brain scans? Brain scans are becoming commonplace as forensic evidence used in courtrooms that, more often than not, mitigate premeditated murder to a lesser offense.

As researchers have shown, prefrontal lobe damage may result in violence, especially in kids who feel like unloved "objects". Predatory parents—parents who physically and emotionally torment their children in ways considered hateful and humiliating—inflict irreparable neurological damage on young, immature nervous systems. Recall that prefrontal lobes comprise the anterior part of the frontal lobes composed of association cortices mediating various *inhibitory controls.* When traumatized, aggression has no behavioral "brakes". But there's more.

Cerebellar, amygdala, and temporal lobe damage exacerbates prefrontal lobe **histopathology.** With devastating cerebral damage, normal sexuality becomes twisted and sexually perverted resulting from addiction to pornography and deviant sexual websites. When rage for being "different" combines with sexual psychopathy, raping and/or murdering unsuspecting victims actually becomes *predictable.*

The expression of serial psychopathy is more about feeling than about cognition. It's more about impulsivity than restraint. It's about expression of pent-up rage in a fractured brain. But, there's more.

In *actus reus,* it is not known precisely why *modus vivendi—the elements of serial crime*—culminate in lashing out and destroying innocence by killing a child or by sexually dominating and controlling a female victim (or in some cases a male victim). However, the *nature of sexual psychopathic crime* is control, domination, and sexual experimentation. Serial killers often go to great lengths to keep the victim alive as long as possible. (Serial killer Jeffrey Dahmer, desperate to preserve a live "sex slave" before his arrest, poured acid into holes he bore in the head of one of his last victims, in a freaky instance of **trephination,** a long abandoned form of "demon" release.)

Horrific psychosocial experiences in dysfunctional milieus (in addition to "cool-coded" brain scans) when compared with other criminals, even those who murder only once, are not the same. Sexual psychopathy produces a serial predator with "lights out" in restraint. Macabre fascination, driven by erotic fantasy, deep in the reptilian brain take over. But, there's more.

That serial killers make a "choice" to commit heinous crime is scientifically untenable. Law enforcement mentality aside, *sexual predators are incapable of making choices like normal people.* Do we expect drug addicts to make choices in the coolness of reason? Is a kid high on "huffing" spray paint making the choice to "huff" when he already suffers from extensive brain damage (not to mention being compelled to "huff" paint by his addiction). Addictionologists remind us that addicts are psychologically and neurologically different than clear-headed individuals. As we have suggested, serial killers are a breed apart; they are *pseudo-sapient,* sexual deviants with damaged brains. They feel "compelled" to rape or kill, due in part to neurological damage from deviant and perverted cognitive maps, and most of all, **poly-addiction** (i.e. pornography, alcohol, cocaine, or other drugs). Because they *feel compelled* by a "brutal urge" they are no less guilty of crimes. They must be incarcerated, or euthanized, as though they had a "choice." They lost choice when they became addicted. They can never be allowed free access to society again. Ever. They are like unsupervised kids in a candy store. But, there's more.

In pornography, depicting females in rape scenes and as willing participants in sadistic sex, anal sex, **fallatio**, and other erotic sexuality fuels the perverse fantasies of sexual psychopaths with a dangerous message: all females are nymphomaniacs and prostitutes—they ask for what they get. Ed Gein sought "specimens" for sexual experimentation to "cure" his sexual repression. But, there's more.

The rapacity of serial crime demonstrates the *profundity* of sexual psychopathy. How could loving, involved parents produce such monstrous pathology in their children? Normal parents don't. Barring brain damage and deviant cognitive mapping from horrific parenting, it's impossible.

Only an unloved child, raised amid the violence of antisocial parenting, is capable of rapacious crime—sadistic torture, evisceration, postmortem slashing, lust/mutilation, satanic, ritualistic crime, pyromania, rape, and pedophilia. An addiction to hardcore, violent pornography, coupled with loveless antisocial parenting, still exists as the single most damaging one-two "punch" of sexual psychopathy.

Developmentally, *lack* of parent-child "contact comfort" through caring, tactile stimulation (touch) produces "contact dissonance," so failure of the associated experience of being held, caressed, loved, and the "nutrient" of motion—being rocked—produces further neurological trauma. But, there's more.

In practical and beneficial ways, youth sports can enhance early (before age 2) parent-child play and also enhance brain activity. Non-contact sports such as gymnastics, swimming, golf, and tennis are especially beneficial. Due to the likelihood of head trauma, football, baseball, soccer, rugby, volleyball, and boxing could exacerbate pre-existing neurological damage with vicious blows to the head. Even the "head butt" in soccer and volleyball can have a cumulative effect in blunt head trauma.

The neurochemistry of rapacious crime involves, to varying degrees, *liberation* of chemistry in the brain (as an agonist) or *suppression* in the brain (as an antagonist) of the following *neurotransmitters,* followed by the principle *emotional feeling* observed in the affective—the *feeling component*—central to serial crime.

1. The liberation of *dopamine* (acting as an agonist) produces the feeling of pleasure, sexual "urges," and eroticism. In sexual psychopathy, deviant cognitive mapping drives the "brutal urge" as elements of *modus*

vivendi, mens rea (the criminal mind), culminating in *actus reus (the criminal act),* and aftermath.

2. The liberation of *norepinephrine* (acting as an agonist) acts as an emotional "focuser" of rapacious behavior equivalent to the "fight or flight" syndrome from fantasy to aftermath.

3. The liberation of *phenylethylamine* (acting as an agonist) produces a jazzed, *erotic rush for a specific physical type* (in organized killers), igniting sexual behavior.

4. The liberation of *testosterone* (acting as an agonist) produces aphrodisiac qualities and sexual drive, as well as aggression—the physical expression of the "brutal urge."

5. By contrast, the *suppression of serotonin* (as an *antagonist*) mitigates the feeling of control. Hence, feeling calm, cool, collected, or confident is supplanted by the "brutal urge"—feeling compelled to act out deviant fantasies. Serotonin (5-HT), an inhibitor of behavior, is the opposite of the "jazzed" focus of norepinephrine (NE).

6. The *suppression* of the hormone *vasopressin* (males) and *oxytocin* (females) blocking feelings associated with social bonding and empathy.

But there's more.

The jurisprudential essence of criminal proceedings has drastically changed in the past few years due to the commanding presence of *neuroscience* in the courtroom. With brain scans in tow, the chance of expert testimony (from forensic neuropsychologists) mitigating first-degree murder to a lesser crime of second-degree murder, or manslaughter, is becoming a reality.

Compelling testimony from forensic pathologists regarding crime scene evidence produces facts. For example, a hair fiber taken from the instrument of death is *forensic fact.* Juries are swayed by fact; facts trump speculative crime reconstruction, traveling in the same orbit with truth. But there's more.

Interestingly, the facts gathered at the crime scene from forensic pathologists are spilling over into expert testimony by neuropsychologists regarding neurological damage in the form of "cool-coded" brain scans. Due to neurological trauma, perpetrators are "compelled" to commit violent crime. Often, first-degree murder, sought by the prosecution, is reduced by the sophisticated brain scans showing "cool-coded" prefrontal lobe damage. To jurors, the sophistication of Positron Emission Tomography (PET), Brain Electrical Activity Mapping (BEAM), Superconducting Interference Device (SQUID), and Magnetic Resonance (MRI) explains the "why"— why he did it. He "did it" due to a neurologically "broken" brain caused by hateful and abusive antisocial parenting. Understanding the ramifications of brain scans, juries are swayed by the neurological sophistication of them. Unless strong counter-arguments are made by experienced forensic neuropsychologists or clinical forensic psychiatrists from the prosecutor's side of the table, the defense "wins" by virtue of mitigation. The client's life is saved from lethal injection. Life in prison is becoming an anticipated verdict when brain scans show "cool-coded" prefrontal lobes.

Vigilance and awareness of the prevalence of serial killers are starting points for preventing family members from being victims of serial crime. To be "vigilant" means to keep "a *vigorous* watch." *Vigorous is the key.*

Parents must be ever aware that serial killers walk freely among us. This fact has to be in the mind of parents anytime their children are outside (even on the front steps) playing.

Serial killers are becoming more arrogant as risk-takers, some grabbing children in plain sight of others, or by coaxing children and teenagers into parked cars. Serial predators may be at children's sporting events, or in parks populated by children at play. They are definitely in, or near, shopping malls. They watch restrooms and convenience stores, or neighborhoods—literally anyplace—where children may not be *vigorously* chaperoned by adults.

They drive through unfamiliar neighborhoods looking for unattended children. They grab and kidnap a child in seconds. Vigilance, not paranoia, is the key. Granted, there is a fine line—a line that can be emotionally exhausting to parents.

There is no such thing as a safe neighborhood anymore. In fact, a safe neighborhood is an oxymoron.

If a serial killer is not roaming free in society, a pedophile or sexual molester may be. Even with Megan's Law, pedophiles still have loopholes.

◼ Sex Offenders & Megan's Law

Sexual molestation is a legal term that centers on *deception and lying* to gain control over a vulnerable victim in a sexually deviant manner. "Deception is the first weapon in the arsenal of a sex offender" so says Jake Goldenflame, a convicted child molester. All molestation is of the same psychological magnitude because physical damage is secondary to the devastating *mental and psychological damage*.

Based on incarceration interviews, most child molesters know their behavior is criminal when they are sexually molesting victims. Even though most offenders feel guilty, the "brutal urge" to seek another victim is greater than feeling of guilt. Some molesters try to *rationalize* their actions as if a personal relationship could exist with the victim. In this way, there behavior is an expression of love.

Like sexual psychopaths, child molesters suffer from neurological dysfunction and chemical imbalances stems from many sources, including horrific parenting and suffering from sexual abuse as a child. In society, a classification of sex offenders exists determined by the severity and the number of crimes committed. *There is no therapeutic cure for sex offenders.* A public notification program called *Megan's law* attempts to alert society to sexual predators.

Megan's Law

On July 29, 1994, Jesse Timmendequas used a puppy to lure Megan Kanka into his home across the street from Megan's residence. He strangled her to unconsciousness with his belt, raped her, asphyxiated her to death with a garbage bag, and discarded her body like a piece of garbage in some bushes only two miles away.

Captured and convicted, he resides on death row in New Jersey for the pernicious murder of Megan Kanka. He was previously convicted of assaulting a child but was released. After her death Megan's Law came into existence *to notify the public that a convicted sex offender was moving into their neighborhood.* Well intentioned, the law has helped, but there exists obvious loopholes. Sexual deviants that are not convicted of serious sex crimes are not put on the list, such as the killer of Polly Klass who's molestation case was plea-bargained by his attorneys to keep him off the public list. (Why, we ask?) In some parts of the country, a fee is attached to access the list no one is allowed to take notes. Typically, sex offenders register and move away without notification. They actively seek to evade the law.

Sex offenders come in all shapes and sizes, therefore, a person's age, weight, or appearance is no indication. You may work, socialize, or attend college with a sex offender and wouldn't even know it. Like serial predators, people with nefarious intention present the opposite demeanor. The dirty old man, hat pulled low over his forehead, naked inside a trench coat, is a dangerous myth.

Student Contributor: Brandon Strickland

Educate Children

Even very young children can be instructed in "stranger danger." A predator trying to snatch a child often does not look like, or talk like, a stranger. They are not hulking creatures dressed in trench coats, a common societal stereotype. Talk show host Oprah Winfrey showed how easy children can be led away by a stranger with a picture of a lost puppy and a dangling leash. *Psychopaths are very crafty manipulators and actors.* They smile or display a pleasant expression when approaching victims. Hence, **subterfuge** is intended to ward off the label of "stranger." If a person approaches a child he or she does not know, running in the opposite direction as soon as possible is the best strategy. Any hesitation may give the intruder the time he needs to grab his next victim.

Sitting nearby and maintaining visual contact with children at play is the best vigilance.

Like Pulling Wisdom Teeth

For adoptive parents, the real challenge is to make children feel safe when abuse issues are suspected from birth parents. It would be wonderful for caring adults to intercept a child headed for psychopathy, but frankly, the odds are against it. As you recall, Jeremy Skotz was adopted into a loving home and later sought out his birth father, a convicted felon, on his own.

Can dysfunctional children ever escape the orbit of deviance?

Ironically, in our blatantly permissive society, teachers and counselors fear being sued by parents; they may have strong suspicions, but must wait to offer assistance until a child is injured or killed. Child Protective Services (CPS) knows the drill very well. Investigators have observed how crafty and dishonest psychopathic parents can be. They roll the dice every time they leave a child with parents who are under CPS investigation.

Loving and nurturing parents talk to their children about everything. By this example, they are encouraging reciprocity from their children. In contrast, antisocial parents spend no time in productive talk; rather they bully and humiliate their children.

The people who should be intervening in children's lives to help with the myriad of adjusts required with everyday problems are the very people that are hatefully preying upon them. By age two, most victims of antisocial parenting are already "lost children."

■ Psychopathy Continuum

According to Robert D. Hare, Ph.D., originator of the *Psychopathy Checklist,* "The one way to appreciate the risks posed by the psychopaths among us is to think of them as predators. *The predator's game is to find and exploit prey.* These social predators often are charming, very convincing, and sometimes fun to be with, but always deceitful and manipulative. In the end, *the victim is the big loser.*"

In our taxonomy, non-criminal psychopathy is indexed *mild* and *moderate,* developing as a consequence of competent, as well as incompetent, parenting. Elsewhere, we have referred to the "mild" and "moderate" variety as "garden variety" psychopaths. However, some "moderate" psychopaths may display criminal behavior in "white collar" crimes.

In *competent parenting* (characterized by love, caring, nurturing, boundaries, and predictability), children may be constantly put on a pedestal and made the center of attention, resulting in *grandiosity of self-worth with narcissistic features* punctuated by "mild" psychopathy. The child behaves as if everyone should cater to his needs, while he is oblivious to the needs of others. This corresponds to the Bowlby (1951) "Type B" bonding, known as *securely attached,* where children display appropriate emotions and resiliency. Egoism aside, they turn out to be terrific kids.

On the other hand, *incompetent parenting,* characterized by *ambivalent* discipline, emotional "distancing," unpredictability, and minimal parenting skills, characterizes the "moderate" version (*psychopathic personality features*) of psychopathy. The development of "moderate" psychopathy may be very close to the criminal variety and may, in fact, produce petty criminals.

In our taxonomy, only hateful, loveless, antisocial (toxic) parenting produces sexual psychopaths (sexual deviates who are criminals) rapists, murderers, and serial killers. More often than not, they display irreversible neurological damage to vital areas of restraint, cognition, and prescient thinking.

The chart on the next page presents our analysis of psychopathy across a behavioral and parental continuum.

Severity of Psychopathy

Mild	Moderate	Severe	Serial Predator
1 Psychopathic Features	2 Psychopathic Personality Features		
6 Incompetent Parenting		3 Antisocial Personality Disorder	5 Sexual Psychopath
		4 Antisocial Parenting	

1→Mild Psychopathy (psychopathic features)

Mild psychopathy can be referred to as "socialized psychopathy"—a non-criminal type. He displays *three or more* psychopathic features from Hare's psychopathy checklist. It includes the "three pillars" of psychopathy—(1) egocentricity, (2) lack of empathy (or care for the suffering of others), and (3) a need to bolster ego through sexual conquests and/or emotional manipulation.

The "mild" psychopath is not a killer or rapist; he may be a successful ladies man or sexual *lothario*. He may be a successful entrepreneur, sports hero, politician, or our favorite relative.

As the "mild" version segues into the "moderate" version, he avoids monogamy by exploiting a variety of sexual partners. He uses sex to bolster self-esteem. He displays a non-criminal *parasitic lifestyle*—living off, or borrowing money from, a string of girlfriends or relatives whom he seldom, if ever, repays. He has authority-figure problems. Developing *psychopathic features* comes from parenting characterized as loving and caring, instilling some discipline and values, yet ambivalence is noted in discipline and affection. A doting mother, who puts her son on a pedestal, and an emotionally absent father create in the son a natural affinity (and a comfort zone) for females due to the constant attention (at first) he gives them.

2→Moderate Psychopathy (psychopathic personality features)

"Moderate" psychopaths display deeper and more profound *psychopathic personality features* marked by "predatory lifestyle" of egocentricity—exaggerated self-confidence, devoid of a conscience or empathy for others, sexual promiscuity, compulsive lying, and blameless and guiltless attitude (even when caught lying or cheating). He displays *five or more* psychopathic characteristics from Hare's psychopathy checklist. This version of psychopathy produces a lack of what some authorities have called "emotional intelligence"—they are superficially glib and display blunt affect (emotionless expression) when discussing a subject matter that one normally expects to see some evidence of emotion (such as the death of a friend or a "sad story").

They live for the moment; they scheme their way into responsible jobs, targeting competitors to manipulate. They adopt their own private agendas for work and relationships. *They use individuals for stimulation and quickly tire of routine.* Fearing exposure and confrontation of their predatory behavior, they often seek out females who do not have fathers in their lives.

3→Antisocial Personality Disorder

DSM Diagnostic Features

According to the DSM, the diagnostic feature of the Antisocial Personality Disorder is *a pervasive pattern of disregard for, and violation of, the rights of others* that begins in childhood or early adolescence and continues into adulthood. The diagnostic criteria (301.7) includes the following:

A. There is a pervasive pattern of disregard for and violation of the rights of others occurring since age 15 years, as indicated by three (or more) of the following:
    1. Failure to conform to social norms with respect to lawful behaviors as indicated by repeatedly performing acts that are grounds for arrest
    2. Deceitfulness, as indicated by repeated lying, use of aliases, or conning others for personal profit or pleasure
    3. Impulsivity, or failure to plan ahead
    4. Irritability and aggressiveness, as indicated by repeated physical fights or assaults
    5. Reckless disregard for safety of self or others
    6. Consistent irresponsibility, as indicated by repeated failure to sustain consistent work behavior or honor financial obligations
    7. Lack of remorse, as indicated by being indifferent to or rationalizing having hurt, mistreated, or stolen from another

B. The individual is at least 18 years of age.

C. There is evidence of *Conduct Disorder* with onset before age 15 years.

D. The occurrence of antisocial behavior is not exclusive during the course of schizophrenia or a manic episode.

Differential Diagnosis

Individuals with *Antisocial Personality Disorder* and *Narcissistic Personality Disorder* share a tendency to be tough-minded, glib, superficial, exploitative, and unsympathetic. In conjunction with the *Histrionic Personality Disorder*, individuals with APD share a tendency to be impulsive, superficial, excitement seekers, reckless, seductive, and manipulative.

Associated Features

Individuals with Antisocial Personality Disorder may display a glib, superficial charm and can be quite *voluble* (talkative) and *verbally facile* (e.g., using technical terms or jargon that might impress someone who is unfamiliar with the topic).

Characteristically, they feel that ordinary work is beneath them, (or lack a realistic concern for their current problems or their future) and may be excessively opinionated, self-assured, or cocky.

They may be irresponsible and exploitative in their sexual relationships. They may have a history of many sexual partners, but may never have sustained a monogamous relationship.

They may experience Dysphoria, including complaints of tension, inability to tolerate boredom, and depressed mood. They may have associated Anxiety Disorders, Depressive Disorders, Substance-Related Disorders, Somatization Disorder, Pathological Gambling, and other disorders of impulsive control.

Child abuse or neglect, unstable or erratic parenting, or inconsistent parental discipline may increase the likelihood that Conduct Disorder will evolve into Antisocial Personality Disorder.

SOURCE: DSM-IV-TR.

4→Antisocial (Toxic) Parenting (aka Netherworld)

In our taxonomy, marked by emotional, physical, and/or sexual abuse, hateful and loveless *antisocial parenting* produces sexual psychopaths. We agree with Bowlby (1951) that children become fearful of parents in this type of parenting. (Type "D") produces *disorganized attachment,* where parents become "frightening to the child". This unsettling condition occurs because of the parent's own traumatic issues. Instead of providing security, parents become an "elicitor of fear" so that children display "anxiety, hostility, and anger". "Cool-coded" brain scans show irreversible neurological brain damage to one or more areas of the brain in children who become sexual psychopaths.

5→Sexual Psychopath

The most severe type of psychopathy is the sexual psychopath, who is a sexual deviant due to horrific antisocial parenting, exacerbated by an addiction to pornography (or sexual repression), and holds an antisocial view of the world.

6→Incompetent Parenting

In our taxonomy, *incompetent parenting,* although at times loving and caring, is characterized by emotional ambivalence and inadequate parenting skills, related to nurturing. (This type of parenting corresponds to John Bowlby's Type "C" *ambivalent/resistant attachment* with "unpredictability of emotional attachment".) Children become "impulsive and helpless" and although normal, they tend to be "clingy" and insecure.

As parents become more hostile to their children and set up conditions where love is withheld, Type "A" *avoidant attachment* is associated with "maternal insensitivity to infant's cues." Infants learn to "distrust parental affection as a defense against being overwhelmed by fear or sadness." "Type A" children tend to "anticipate rejection and become hostile or angry." Due to the anger issues, psychopathic personality features of "moderate" psychopathy characterize aspects of this parental agenda.

As a society, we cannot expect a better class of citizens without a better class of parents. As we stated in an earlier chapter, this book is about the causes of psychopathy—horrific parenting exacerbated by a pornography compulsion, poly-addiction, and brain trauma—observed through effects—unsuspecting victims being destroyed, preyed upon pseudo-sapient predator.

In the final analysis, no ideology, science, philosophy, or system of behavioral analysis—religion, spirituality, psychology, sociology, criminology, medicine, psychiatry, nothing exists to "save" or provide a way to turn around sexual psychopathy.

Not yet, that is.

The focus of religion and spirituality is sin, or more correctly, how to fill the void in one's life by "filling" our heart and mind with the Holy Spirit or oneness with the cosmos. Both ask us to dedicate ourselves to a higher calling. The religions of the world seek union with a creator, God, while spirituality seeks unity to a grand scheme of love and appreciation of life in all its forms. *The sexual psychopath is too sick to embrace such higher callings.*

Psychology focuses on the uniqueness and individuality of the person as he grapples with *intrapsychic* forces—within himself and *interpsychic* forces—outside factors related to the dynamic interaction with others and the demands of society. He seeks *homeostatis,* a healthy balance. *The severely chemically imbalanced mind of sexual psychopaths is the very antithesis of homeostatis.*

Sociology seeks to understand how the group, the family, and the "tribe" alters or modifies behavior in the concrete "jungles" of modern society. Sociology can only describe and document the devastation of anti-social families.

Medicine and psychiatry seek the eradication of diseases that cripple and psychologically maim. Is there a Prozac® on the horizon for psychopathy?

Philosophy—the oldest of the "sciences"—seeks to assuage anxiety though knowledge, the word itself means "love (*philo*) of knowledge (*sophia*). Knowledge leads to understanding and peace of mind, something that cannot be envisioned by sexual predators. All the aforementioned seek to help, to give individuals more insight than they had, to enrich, and to inspire!

◾ The Mark of the Beast

Neurophysics

As we have seen, the sexual psychopath seeks the antithesis of life. He butchers life. He seeks to take away all we have. *In his nihilism, he is a destroyer.* Therefore, no ideology, or system of knowledge, currently exists to offer "salvation," or a way out, or a "way to make it better" for sexual predators. The only hope may come from an unlikely science, and from an unlikely industry. The science is *physics,* or rather, **QM (quantum mechanics)** as applied to computer chip technology. QM is the theory that "allows us to design postage stamp-size computers that do billions of calculations in a second, and to build nuclear weapons." Applying QM to computer chips, "neurophysicists" may one day provide a "bionic brain" chip for damaged pseudo-sapient brains, not only for sexual predators, but for all those suffering from severe psychiatric illnesses—clinical depression, paranoid schizophrenia, bipolarity, and DID (dissociative identity disorder)—all those for which psychotropic medications have failed. *Perhaps, the "mark of the beast" will be some outward sign—an indelible inscription or some other identifying mark, perhaps on his/her forehead— telling the world that the person whose outer persona we perceive has an implanted microchip regulating electrical impulses to a fractured brain.* The microchip runs on a tiny lithium battery with a charging circuit activated by changes in skin temperature. Reportedly, "almost two million dollars was spent finding the two places in the body that the temperature changes the most rapidly—in the forehead and on the back of the hand." (The same two places mentioned in Revelation.)

If psychoparmacology from "Prozac Nation" can't help, maybe "neurophysics"—a discipline whose time may have arrived—can and will reverse sexual psychopathy and relieve the world of sexual predators. *The metaphor of "666" is just too tempting to translate (somewhat tongue-in-cheek) as psycho . . . pathic . . . killer—each word containing 6 letters. Time will tell.*

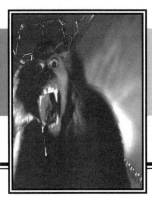

Aftermath

I. Word Scholar

Define the following words from *The Word Scholar Glossary*.

1. Flat affect _____

2. Poly-addiction _____

3. Fallacio _____

4. Megan's Law _____

5. "Mild" psychopathy _____

6. "Moderate" psychopathy _____

7. Incompetent parenting _____

8. Neurophysics _____

9. Quantum mechanics (QM) _____

10. "Bionic" brain _____

II. The Forensic Lab

Compose a one page report addressing: When "bionic brain" computer chip technology arrives to repair the damaged brains of sexual psychopaths (we speculate within 10 years), what identifiers, if any, such as a glowing red bionic eye, or a new "Scarlet Letter" worn at all times should alert Homo sapiens the person standing in front of them was a former pseudo-sapien sexual predator? What happens to the manufacturer when the unit malfunctions?

Epilog

▪ Five Parental Nurturing Skills

Courtesy of criminal profiling students, intent upon preventing the development of a child with a psychopathic personality disorder or sexual psychopathy, we provide five salient parenting skills that are the antithesis of antisocial parenting.

1. Be in love with the idea of having your children, or take responsible precautions (not the "rhythm method"*) not to get pregnant in the first place (Males are you listening!). Hug, kiss, hold, touch and comfort your children. (Find a sturdy rocking chair and use it to age two, at least). Provide the best financial support possible. Money CAN buy happiness and a normal childhood. *Every child deserves a carefree, fun childhood.*

2. Take time. Communicate with your children. Be involved in their school experiences. Spend quality time in play. Mothers, read to your children while they are still in the womb. Let them hear you laugh often before and after birth.

3. Listen. Listen some more. Encourage your children in new endeavors. Be understanding and patient. When you're nerves get frayed, let your spouse take over. Show emotional support for the family unit. Everyone has "a place" in family. Respect everyone's place—sense of belonging and contributions.

4. Provide a stable home life with predictability, discipline, and boundaries. Never *enable* your children to continue to "act out" or misbehave by reinforcing dysfunctional patterns. You know what's right and wrong. Ethics is no more than good, practical, commonsense parenting. Stop and smell the roses with your children.

5. Laugh some more. Have fun with your children. Have big birthday parties. Open your home to your children's friends. Don't be embarrassed by any subject your child brings up. You're both a parent and a teacher to your child for the rest of your life. Model good-hearted behavior. Kiss them good night as long as you want to. Before you turn out the light, take a lingering look at the miracle that's in your hands and up to you to mold.

---

*The "rhythm method" explains how many females get pregnant, although it is intended to be *prophylactic*. Avoiding birth control tablets (because it makes her sick or causes weight gain), and knowing her boyfriend hates condoms (because it reduces feeling), she tries to predict (roughly) the exact time of ovulation in her monthly cycle. She avoids having sex around that time. She attempts to get into her cyclical "rhythm". No egg, no pregnancy, no problem. Right? Wrong. Viable sperm "live" in the female reproductive tract four to five days, sometimes up to a week. So, the "rhythm method" is a fallacy and produces pregnancy.

◼ The Building Blocks of Sexual Psychopathy

1. Antisocial Parenting

Hateful and loveless antisocial parenting forges the foundation and *developmental* component for sexual predators. Severely dysfunctional homes produce children and adolescents full of rage for being abused, neglected, or unloved. However, some children overcome the worst possible parenting due to some unknown resiliency to become high achievers. *Antisocial parenting alone does not make a sexual predator.*

2. Brain Damage

As the *neurological component* of sexual psychopathy, neurological damage to one or more of the soft cortical tissue of the brain associated with prescient thinking, consequences, remorsefulness, rationality, or "anger management" can be devastating and diverse. Prefrontal lobe damage reflects what we attribute as personality or "self in relation to the world." Prefrontal lobes are involved in complex cognitive "choices" of appropriate versus inappropriate behavior. Additionally, damage to temporal lobes, amygdala, or cerebellum produce a brain that, ironically, is "programmed" for sexual predatory behavior, giving the "green light" to reptilian cortices.

3. Pornography Obsession or Sexual Repression

The deviant *cognitive scripting component* develops perverted cognitive mapping is the obsessional thinking and compulsive (behavior) surrounding pornography (or in the alternative, the repression of sexuality) resulting in the *format and focus* of perverted thinking (or morbid curiosity), and the anticipated "thrilling high" of controlling and dominating females (and/or children) in sexual "slavery." Cognition "merges" with feeling by way of cognitive scripting and neurochemistry to produce sexualized thinking from erotic sources.

4. Deviant Cognitive Mapping

This accounts for the *perceptional component*—the sexually perverted way of looking at females, children (and males). The foregoing components produce the neurochemical "mindset" of the sexual pyschopaths so that *feelings* from normal brain chemistry and hormones become "attached" to perverted sexuality and thinking so that sexual predators feel *compelled* to commit crime due to addiction.

5. Poly-Addiction

The all important *addiction component* exemplifies addicted to their own brain chemistry for the "thrilling high" of sexual domination and control of helpless or unsuspecting victims. Sexual predators are addicted to the "feeling" produced by their own DA, NE, PEA, 5-HT, GABA, and testosterone.

In Summation

In sexual psychopathy, developmental, neurological, cognitive scripting, perception, and addiction components exists in sexual psychopathy for which there is no return to normalcy.

Word Scholar Glossary

A

Ach (acetylcholine) (ugh-see-tull-co-leen)
Ubiquitous neurotransmitter and parasympathetic agent, Ach is responsible for conservation of energy, attention and memory, thirst, sex, mood, REM sleep, and is present at muscle receptors for muscle contraction.

ADD (attention-deficit disorder)
A common learning disorder of inattention and lack of focus affecting mostly males.

ADHD (attention-deficit hyperactivity disorder)
A common learning disorder of inattention with a hyperactive component affecting mostly males.

aberrant (ab-er-unt)
Literally, "to go astray;" atypical behavior or thinking.

actus reus (act-us ray-us)
Literally, "criminal act;" the physical part of a crime.

addiction
Pertains to a compulsive need for a habit-forming substance to produce a feeling state that "compels" the user to continue. Addiction is more about the feeling it produces and the desire to replicate the feeling.

addictionology
The science of addiction related to substance abuse, tolerance, psychophysiological habituation, and neurochemistry of addiction.

adrenaline
Powerful hormone secreted by the adrenal glands related to fight or flight.

affective (AF-ekk-tive)
Pertains to feelings; contrast affect ("feeling") with *cognitive* ("thinking").

agonist (AG-un-st)
A chemical substance capable of combining with a receptor, liberating the targeted substance.

amygdala (ugh-mig-dugh-lugh)
Limbic system structure of gray matter in the anterior temporal lobe, center of emotional memory and aggression.

analgesic (anal-jee-sik)
Literally, "insensitivity to pain."

androgenic (and-dr-gen-ik)
Pertains to the action of the powerful male sex hormone testosterone.

anecdotal (ann-ik-dough-tul)
Literally "unpublished." Refers to a short narrative or story of real life experiences.

anhedonia (ann-ugh-doan-ee-uh)
Experiencing displeasure.

anima (ann-ugh-mugh)
Refers to Carl G. Jung's analytic theory of the archetypes of masculinity and femininity. Literally "soul"—pertains to the feminine part of a male's personality.

animism (ann-ugh-miz-um)
The belief that spirits occupies all things and influence outcomes.

animus (ann-ugh-muss)
Refers to Carl G. Jung's analytic theory of archetypes of masculinity and femininity. Literally, "courage"—pertains to the masculine part of a female's personality.

antecedent (ann-tugh-see-dunt)
Pertains to former events as shaping current behavior or conditions.

antisocial developmental programming
Refers to the slow, stage-by-stage, effect of detrimental influences contributing to psychopathic personality such as antisocial parenting. May include a combination of physical, sexual, or verbal abuse, pornography, drug abuse, or other factors leading to full-blown psychopathic behavior with a pronounced feeling of isolation, emotional disconnectedness, and inability to bond, or feel love.

antisocial parenting
Pertains to the most damaging and destructive type of loveless and hateful parenting most often observed in the development of sexual psychopathy. Antisocial parenting is characterized by a combination of physical, sexual, and/or verbal abuse, alcoholism, poly-drug abuse, where compulsive viewing of pornography, prostitution, and spousal abuse occur routinely.

antisocial personality disorder
In the DSM, a pervasive pattern of disregard for, and violation of, the rights of others that begins in childhood or early adolescence and continues into adulthood.

anxiety
Characterized as a fearful concern or uneasiness of mind due to the imbalance of GABA, a neurotransmitter.

aphorism (AF-ugh-riz-um)
Literally, "to define." A concise statement of a principle or sentiment.

aphrodisiac (aff-roe-dee-zee-ak)
A sexual stimulant; a substance that arouses sexual desire.

apocalyptical (ugh-pok-ugh-lip-tee-kul)
Prophetic; foreboding imminent disaster.

archetype (ARK-type)
Refers to a perfect example or a specimen, an inherited idea in the analytic psychology of Carl G. Jung derived from the experiences of the race and is present in the unconscious of the individual such as anima and animus.

assessment
Literally "to sit beside" another, refers to making a psychological appraisal of another who is "up close and personal."

association cortices (cor-tugh-seez)
Loosely referred to as cognition; comprising most of the cerebral surface of the human brain responsible for complex processing between the arrival of input and the generation of behavior.

autoerotic (augh-toe-erot-ik)
sexual self-stimulation; masturbation

autoerotic asphyxiation (azz-fix-ee-a-shun)
Refers to the practice of reducing oxygen to the brain through self-strangulation (often by hanging) accompanied by masturbation. Intensifying orgasm is the goal behind this dangerous practice that can lead to accidental death.

B

behaviorism (also known as behavioral psychology)
The study of *observable behavior* without regard to cognition or affective (feeling) states, which are considered introspective tools and not scientifically valid or reliable.

blocking reuptake
Pertains to a chemical antagonist preventing neurochemical reclamation of molecules of neurotransmitters back into axonal vesicles.

body language
Refers to non-verbal body "language" such as tone of voice, facial expression, or posturing.

borderline personality disorder (or borderline features)
In the DSM, a disorder characterized by severe distortions of self-image, mood, and interpersonal relations. "Borderlines" experience marked mood shifts, impulsivity, difficulty tolerating loneliness, and are emotionally needy typified by pronounced fear of abandonment.

brain stem
Portion of the brain that lies between the diencephalon and spinal cord; comprises the midbrain, pons, and medulla.

British empiricism
Chiefly due to John Locke's influence upon philosophy, the intellectual climate (zeitgeist) of North America moved more rapidly toward association of experiences as causes of behavior influencing the study of psychology. Psychology "turned the corner" away from philosophy toward behavioral explanations with British empiricism.

C

CNS (central nervous system)
Pertains to the brain and spinal cord.

CPS (child protective service)
A state child advocacy agency aimed at preventing child abuse or interceding on a child's behalf when abuse is proven.

catecholamines (cat-ugh-coal-ugh-means)
Neurotransmitter amines (chemical compound containing one or more halogen atoms attached to nitrogen) related to catachol, namely norepinephrine and dopamine.

catharsis (or **cathartic**) (kugh-thor-sis)
Purging of emotions (such as anger, guilt) through discourse with a therapist (or trusted friend); literally, "talk therapy."

cerebellum (sara-bell-um)
Prominent hindbrain structure characterized by motor coordination, posture, and balance.

chaining
Behavioral term relating to sequencing of behavior where small muscular movements are learned and "chained" together producing a desired action, such as behavior required to hit a baseball.

classical conditioning
Behavioral paradigm characterized by the law of association where one stimulus (the unconditioned stimulus—UCS) is paired with another, a formerly neutral stimulus, to produce a new behavioral contingency, the conditioned stimulus—CS. Through association, the bell (CS) came to stand for the original stimulus (the food—the UCS) in Pavlov's famous experiment.

co-dependency
A psychological condition where a person is controlled or manipulated by another person with a pathological condition such as addiction, obsessive-compulsive personality disorder, or psychopathy.

cognitive
Refers to "thinking".

cognitive-behavioral perspective
Specialty within general psychology focusing on how cognition (thinking) influences behavior, especially in forming powerful "cognitive maps" of learning and thinking. Also referred to as "soft" behaviorism.

cognitive mapping
Powerful thinking "maps" of experience which affect behavior in far-reaching and profound ways.

cognitive neuroscience
Neuropsychological specialty that deciphers the structural and functional organization of specific brain regions connected to cognition by case studies of neurological patients, the advent of noninvasive brain imaging, and primate studies.

cognitive psychology
Psychological specialty that seeks to understand the psychophysiological process of thinking and how thought processes impact behavior.

collective unconscious
Jungian concept related to a genetically shared unconscious by all members of a race or ethnicity.

colloquial (cugh-low-qwe-ull)
Used in conversation; non-technical words and/or expressions.

concussion
A potentially serious head injury where the soft tissue of the brain is violently jarred against the bony cranium.

contusion
A serious head injury that results in bruising, bleeding, and trauma to the brain.

compliant co-offender
Refers to a compliant person "recruited" by an offender.

compulsion
An irresistible impulse to perform an irrational act.

conduct disorder
In the DSM, refers to a repetitive and persistent pattern of behavior in which the basic rights of others or major age-appropriate societal norms or rules are violated.

conflict theory
Freudian theory relative to cross-purposes of id, ego, and superego with resulting anxiety.

consumerism
Marketing of consumer goods to increase consumption.

continuum
A line denoting possible causes or answers to given questions in behavioral science.

"cool-coded"
Refers to blue colored ("cool-coded") brain scans (according to Jacobs) of neurologically damaged individuals in brain areas such as the prefrontal lobes. In undamaged brains the scans glow pink or red indicating normal blood flow.

corpus delicti (cor-pus dugh-lek-teye)
Refers to the *body of evidence* required to prove a crime was committed such as mens rea—the mental part, actus reus—the physical part, and the dead body of the victim.

cri de coeur (kree-dugh-coor)
Literally, passionate "cry from the heart."

criminologist
One who studies crime as a social phenomenon, criminal activity and behavior, and incarceration variables.

cynicism
Contemptuously distrustful of human nature; a sneering disbelief in sincerity.

D

DID (Dissociative Identity Disorder)
In the DSM, a serious mental disorder related to multiple identities residing within the same person, formerly referred to as Multiple Personality Disorder (MPD).

DSM (Diagnostic and Statistical Manual of Mental Disorders)
Diagnostic and descriptive "textbook" of mental disorders used by mental health professionals such as clinical psychologists and psychiatrists.

decadence (deck-ugh-dunce)
Marked by decline and deterioration.

deductive
Pertains to speculative logic or "hunches" (termed *a priori* reasoning in philosophy), where no systematized knowledge exists as a yardstick to measure present or future behavior. Contrast *inductive*, the logic of science, the opposite of deductive.

deny (denial)
Freudian defense against anxiety where the person consciously disclaims the importance of an issue. Contrast to repression which operates as "unconscious denial."

dependent personality disorder
Characterized by a passive, "clingy," submission to others; a "doormat" personality with separation anxiety and fear. A compliant co-offender often has a full-blown dependent personality disorder.

developmental psychology
Psychological specialty that studies stages or periods of physical and psychological development and corresponding expectations across the lifespan.

dimorphic nuclei (die-mor-fick)
An identifiable part of the anterior hypothalamus show male/female differentiation.

dissonant (diss-ugh-nunce)
Pertains to insufficiency of agreement resulting in lack of consonance.

dopamine (DA) (dopa-meen)
A powerful neurotransmitter known to lie behind pleasure across a wide continuum.

dogma
Presented as authoritative or established opinion without adequate grounds.

dualism
A view that human beings are composed of two irreducible elements—matter and spirit.

dual diagnosis
A diagnosis made when a chemical dependency exists alongside a pure psychopathology such as depression or anxiety.

E

efficacy (F-ugh-kugh-see)
Power to produce an effect such as truth.

egocentric
Limited to outlook or interest to one's own activities; self-centered and egotistical.

emitted behavior
Pertains to everyday behavior occurring due to no identifiable stimulus, a subject of operant conditioning.

empiricism (em-peer-ugh-ciz-um)
Refers to laboratory analysis and reporting, objectivity, observation, and replication of studies in experimental psychology.

enabler
One who helps another to persist in self-destructive behavior.

enuresis (In-yur-ree-sis)
Pertains to bed-wetting.

environmental psychology
Concerned with influences of the environment—neighborhoods, noise and congestion, and employment—and how these influences affect behavior.

epiphany (ugh-piff-ugh-nee)
Pertains to an illuminating discovery or insight.

eroticism
Pictorial, literary, or graphic portraying sexual desire or sexual themes.

esoteric (S-ugh-ter-ik)
Literally "within". Refers to being understood by a specially initiated person.

ethnocentrism (Eth-no-sin-tris-um)
Pertains to race and characterized by the belief that one's own racial group is superior to all others.

etiology (E-T-ology)
Refers to causation.

evisceration (ee-viss-err-ra-shun)
To disembowel; remove the entrails of another.

evolutionary neuroanatomy
Neuropsychological analysis of the evolution of the brain into three layers—reptilian, "old mammalian," and neo-cortex for purposes of delineation of neuroanatomy and concomitant neurochemical influences.

exacerbate (ig-saz-sir-bate)
To make worse.

excitement phase
In Masters and Johnson's human sexual response, the first stage of sexual excitement prompted by erotic thoughts, sights, or contact.

existential (Egg-sugh-stin-shul)
Grounded in the experience of being or existing.

exorcism
In Catholicism, to expel Satan or an evil spirit.

extrapolate
To project or extend known data into an unknown area so the use of *conjecture* guides the way.

extravert
Refers to a "people person"—a gregarious and unreserved individual who seeks people and people-orientated activities to feel jazzed.

F

fait accompli (Fate-ugh-comp-lee)
Literally, "the accomplished fact."

fellatio (fuh-LAY-she-oh)
Stimulation of the penis by the mouth.

fetish
Sexual arousal caused by objects (high-heeled shoe) or body parts.

flat affect
Emotionless.

forensic neuropsychologist
A specialist (and often an expert witness) within neuropsychology who presents courtroom testimony (often in the form of brain scans) in criminal cases related to potential causes of criminality from medical sources such as neurology, biology, and brain scanning technology.

forensic pathologist
An MD-trained physician who analyzes pathology such as cause of death and related issues from autopsy protocols that are headed to the courtroom.

forensic psychologist
A Ph.D.-trained psychologist who testifies in court as an expert witness regarding sanity or insanity, or pathological issues of a given participant.

forensic science
Pertains to the science of criminal evidence gathering by forensic pathologists, who often testify in a courtroom.

frontal lobes
The largest of four lobes of the brain with a wide repertoire of functions including cognition.

frottage (fr-ugh-tah-jh)
Secretly rubbing against another for sexual pleasure or fantasizing a caring relationship.

futurist
A journalist or intellectual who writes or speculates about the future.

G

GABA (Gamma-aminobutyric acid)
Found primarily in the hippocampus, hypothalamus, and amygdala, a powerful inhibitory neurotransmitter that reduces arousal, aggression, and anxiety.

garrote (gugh-rott)
Pertains to a device or a noose used in strangulation.

glib
Literally, "slippery"; marked by ease and informality; nonchalant.

glutamate
The major excitatory neurotransmitter in the CNS believed to underlie all learning thought synaptic cleft sequencing.

H

hard core porn
Refers to pornographic pictures, material, or any visual manifestation of explicit and often times deviant sexual behavior usually rated as XXX.

the hawthorne effect
Refers to Elton Mayo's famous field study showing the mere fact of being observed stimulates output or achievement.

hedonistic (He-dun-is-tik) **hedonism**
Pleasure-seeker.

hemispherectomy (HIM-us-fear-reck-tugh -me)
Removal of one or both cerebral hemispheres.

hippocampus (hippo-camp-us)
A cortical structure in the medial portion of the temporal lobe; in humans the center for learning and short term declarative memory.

histopathy (hist-op-ugh-thee)
Branch of physiology concerned with tissue changes characteristic of pathology.

histrionic (histrionic personality features)
(Usually a female) who acts dramatic and theatrical for affect.

holistic (holism)
Concerned with complete systems rather than dissection into parts.

homicidal triad
Refers to bed wetting at an inappropriate age, setting fires, and violence against peers or pets as precursors to severe conduct disorder showing lack of control.

hubris (hew-bris)
Exaggerated pride or self-confidence.

humanism (humanistic psychology)
Focus on human interests and values.

hypocrisy
Pertains to presenting a false appearance of virtue

hypothalamus
A collection of nuclei in the diencephalon governing reproduction, homeostatis, and circadian rhythm.

I

I/O Psychology
Refers to Industrial/Organizational Psychology, a specialty of applying psychological principles to business and industry.

id
Pertains to the biological inheritance of "mind" or "personality" as instincts of a sexual and aggressive nature from Freud's psychoanalytic school.

idiosyncratic (id-e-oh-sin-krad-ik)
Pertains to the uniqueness of an individual.

inductive (IN-duc-tive)
Pertains to the methodology of science. Inductive logic is termed *a posteriori* reasoning in philosophy, where systematized knowledge is used (such as *known offender characteristics* in criminal profiling) as a yardstick in analyzing present and future behavior. The opposite of inductive is deductive, or speculative logic used by Sherlock Holmes as "elementary observation."

ignominious (igg-non-ugh-muss)
Dishonorable, despicable.

in loco parentis (N-loco-pugh-ren-tus)
A legal term meaning "in the place of the parents."

incompetent parenting
Pertains to ambivalence in parenting—withholding love, inconsistent punishment, inattentiveness, and lack of adequate nurturing skills that produce children who may seek therapy later in their lives.

intellectualize
Freudian defense against anxiety where the person verbalizes elaborate excuses without addressing feelings.

internal dialogue
Refers to "talking" or thinking to oneself.

intrapsychic (N-trugh-sigh-kick)
Literally "inside one's head" as might occur in internal dialogue.

internal locus of control (ILOC)
Refers to social learning theorist Julian Rotter's theory of expectations. Internal LOC refers to a responsible person who trusts his plan or strategy for success accomplished by hard work. (Contrast External Locus of Control where luck or timing controls one's expectations of the future).

introvert
Pertains to a type of personality marked by robust intrapsychic activity so that territoriality and time alone are valued over the "people person" who seeks additional social interaction.

inventory test
Refers to any of a number of standard personality tests.

L

LSD (lysergic acid diethylamide)
Pertains to a chemical substance that produces vivid hallucinatory (psychedelic) experiences.

law of association
In behavioral psychology, the law that states when two stimuli are paired together in time, one (the conditioned stimulus—the CS) comes to stand for the other, or the natural stimulus—the UCS. UCS is natural while CS is learned.

law of effect
In behavioral psychology, the famous law proposed by Edward Thorndike stating that behavior increases when followed by "satisfiers" and decreases when followed by "annoyers." Precursor law to operant condition.

law of frequency
In behavioral psychology, the law that states the more frequently we perform a certain behavior the more likely we will continue it in the future; literally practice makes perfect.

law of recency
In behavioral psychology, the law that states the more recently we performed a certain behavior the more likely we will continue to perform it in the future.

Lesch-Nyhan Syndrome (LNS)
A rare and usually fatal genetic disorder transmitted as a recessive trait on the X chromosome. LNS is characterized by hyperuricemia (excessive uric acid), spasticity, rigidity, and compulsive biting of the lips and fingers caused by an absence of the HPRT enzyme and the resulting damage to the midbrain.

libido (lugh-bee-doe)
The sex drive.

learned helplessness
Pertains to a condition when a person feels helpless when he encounters conditions over which he has no prior experience or control.

litigious (lugh-tee-jus)
Pertains to law suits.

lothario
A seducer of women.

lycanthropy (LIE-can-throw-pee)
A psychiatric condition in mind only where a patient imagines himself to be a wolf.

M

MFB (medial forebrain bundle)
Pertains to the medial forebrain bundle of the hypothalamus, dubbed the "pleasure pathway" due to prevalence of dopamine receptors.

macabre (mugh-cob)
Morbid preoccupation and fascination with death or thoughts of death.

magical thinking
Pertains to psychotic episodes where patients feel their thinking produces precognitive or paranormal events that defy the physical world.

manie sans delire
Literally, "obsession without insanity," which later becomes the basis of psychopathic personality.

malum in se
Literally "evil in itself." Pertains to serious crimes against personal safety in criminal law such as murder or rape.

masochism (maz-ugh-kism) **masochist**
A sexual deviation characterized by the enjoyment of having pain inflicted.

munchausen syndrome by proxy
Deliberately making another person sick evidently for attention and pity. Also known as Factitious Disorder by proxy.

mass murderer
Pertains (usually) to a male killer who kills four or more people in one incident, in one location, and in one emotional experience.

Megan's law

Law intended to protect citizens against sexual offenders came into affect on October 31, 1994. The New Jersey State Legislature enacted the law requiring certain convicted sexual offenders to register with law enforcement providing community notification of sex offenders.

melatonin (mel-ugh-tone-un)

Powerful hormone secreted by the pineal gland involved in the sleep-wake cycle. Implicated in the depressive disorder SAD (seasonal affective disorder).

metencephalon (met-in-sef-ugh-lin)

One of the six divisions of the brain; pertains to the pons and the cerebellum.

mens rea (menz ray-ugh)

Literally "criminal mind."

milieu (mill-you).

Refers to a social context, such as family, school, or peers where learning and experiences occur

modus vivendi (MO-dus Vugh-vin-dee)

According to Jacobs (2003), the five components of sexualized serial crime including *mens rea, actus rea, modus operandi,* signature, and aftermath.

"morally fuzzy"

Pertains to popular semantics where meaning is defined from the perspective of the speaker. How "spin" controls meaning.

morphology

Pertains to the body or body type.

motive

Literally, "to move." Emotion or desire acting on will; motivation.

medulla oblongata (mugh-do-lugh-Ob-lun-got-ugh)

The most caudal of the brain stem serving sensory and motor systems including involuntary "automatic" actions such as heart rate and blood pressure.

mesencephalon (mez-in-sef-ugh-lun)

Pertains to midbrain structures of the red nucleus and substantia nigra involving movement.

mullerian ducts

Tiny microscopic ducts that determine internal and external female genitalia.

multiaxial system

Refers to domains of patient information reviewed by clinicians in clinical psychology.

myelencephalon (meye-in-sef-ugh-lun)

Refers to the medulla or medulla oblongata.

myelinized (My-lun-eye-zd)

The process of axonal insulation by a white fatty substance known as myelin.

N

narcissistic personality disorder
In the DSM, a pervasive personality disorder characterized by egocentrism. Often observed in conjunction with psychopathic personality characteristics.

narcissism
Literally "self-love.'

nature
Refers to biological inheritance. Contrast to nurture, or social learning.

necrophilia (neck-row-feel-ee-ugh)
A sexual perversion marked by an obsession with having sex with a corpse.

nefarious (nu-fair-ee-us)
Flagrantly wicked.

neocortex
Literally "new bark." Refers to the micro-thin, most recently evolved part on the upper-most part of the brain.

neoplasm
Literally "tumor."

netherworld
Literally "underworld." Pertains to a counter-culture of antisocial parenting that produces sexual psychopaths.

neurology
The medical specialty and scientific study of the nervous systems of the body in regard to structure, function, and abnormalities.

neuropeptide
An endogenous chain of proteins (peptides) that influences neural activity.

neurophysics
Proposed by Jacobs (2003) as the science responsible for merging quantum theory with computer chip technology thereby developing a "bionic brain" transplant to correct diseased or pathological cortices in the brain due to disease, trauma, or neglect.

neuropsych paradigm
Pertains to the central importance of neurotransmitters and neurohormones that give rise to thinking, behavior and personality—ultimately normal versus abnormal, and criminal behavior.

neuropsycholinguists
The neuropsych specialty that studies how word knowledge and usage changes brain chemistry and behavior.

neuropsychology (new-row-sigh-kol-ogy) **neuroscientist**
Psychological specialization that merges psychology, neurology, and neurochemistry to study underpinnings of behavior at the tissue level of interneurons.

neuro-psych-bio-social perspective
Pertains to an eclectic perspective of systematized knowledge and influences from neurology, psychology, biology, and sociology in a comprehensive analysis of behavior.

neurotheologist (neurotheology)
Pertains to biological basis observable in brain scans producing euphoria for spiritual or mystical experiences.

nihilist (nigh'l-ist)
Belief that society is so corrupt that traditional values, moral truths, or beliefs are unfounded and that existence is senseless and useless

norepinephrine (NE)
Neurotransmitter acting as a "focuser" of "jazzed" activities.

nosology (noz-oll-ugh-gee)
Refers to a classification of diseases.

nurture
Refers to care of others in social learning, contrasted to *nature* or biological inheritance.

nymphomania
Literally "inner lips of the vulva". Excessive sexual desire by a female.

O

ODD (oppositional defiant disorder)
In the DSM, a pervasive behavioral disorder of opposition to authority displayed by adolescents.

obsession
A persistent disturbing preoccupation with an often unreasonable idea or feeling; compelling motivation.

obsessive-compulsive
Pertains to persistence in thinking (obsession) and action (compulsion). Rigidity of thinking and doing exemplified as "my way or the highway".

obsessive-compulsive disorder
In the DSM, a psychological disorder related to rigid behavior characterized by routine and protocol, termed "anal retentive" by Freud.

operant conditioning
In behaviorism, a form of learning characterized by consequences or "payoffs" where behavior is shaped and maintained by positive and negative consequences.

operant (OP-er-unt)
In behaviorism, any behavior capable of being reinforced.

operational definition
Pertains to defining terms used in intellectual discourse so participants are on the same page.

orgasmic phase
> The summit of Master and Johnson's human sexual response characterized by orgasm—ejaculation and release of muscular tension.

overkill
> Pertains to excessive brutality in *actus reus* phase of *modus vivendi,* such as 50 stab wounds perpetrated on the victim, when one wound could have brought death.

oxytocin (OXY)
> Powerful hormone known as the "cuddle chemical" related to social bonding.

P

PEA (phenylethylamine) (Fugh-neth-lugh-meen)
> An endogenous amine similar to methamphetamine responsible for the "romantic" rush of physical attraction.

PMS (premenstrual syndrome)
> Denotes mood changes and other emotional and physical discomforts just prior to the menstrual period.

PNS (peripheral nervous system)
> Refers to the portion of the nervous system outside the brain and spinal cord such as the somatic and autonomic systems.

PTSD (post-traumatic stress disorder)
> Denotes an enduring, distressful emotional disorder that follows exposure to a severe fear-inducing threat.

pan-hedonism
> Literally "all sexual".

paranoia
> Literally "demented mind". Denotes a psychosis characterized by systematic delusions (false beliefs) of grandeur or persecution.

paranoid
> Overly suspicious or fearful.

Parkinson's disease
> A chronic movement disorder characterized by jerky movements and muscle rigidity.

paradigm (para-dime)
> A framework for presentation of systematic or scientific ideas or concepts.

paraphilia
> Literally "abnormal love." Refers to unusual sexual practices or special erotic activities that may victimize non-consenting persons such as voyeurism or exhibitionism.

pedophilia (ped-ugh-feely-ugh) (pedophile) (ped-ugh-file)
> Sexual perversion in which children are preferred sexual objects.

pejorative (pugh-jar-ugh-tive)
Having a negative connotation.

perception
How a person organizes sensation. Pertains to one's view of reality or any subset through physical sensation.

personality disorder
In the DSM, characteristic behavior listed taxonomically with the most salient presenting symptoms of a variety of personality disorders, such as antisocial personality disorder, the most frequent personality disorder observed in psychopathy.

personality disorder NOS (PD NOS)
In the DSM, a personality disorder category with features of more than one personality disorder so that a person diagnosed PD NOS may display narcissism along with antisocial personality.

persona
Literally, "social mask". The many social demeanors expressed by a single individual.

personation
Pertains to a killer's signature.

phenomenology (fugh-nom-ugh-noll-ugh-gee)
Refers to phenomena that make up conscious experiences and self-awareness.

physiological psychology
Refers to experimental psychology and the interaction of body-brain.

picquerist (pick-er-ist)
Refers to a killer who is sexually stimulated by penetrating the skin with knife cuts or wounds.

plateau phase
In Masters and Johnson's human sexual response, the psychophysiological experience and feeling that sex is imminent.

pleasure principle
Denotes Freudian concept of the role of fantasy within libido (or sex drive).

pluripotent (plur-rip-ugh-tent)
Refers to developmental plasticity.

poly-addiction
Addiction to more than one chemical substance.

pontine tegmentum (pon-teen teg-men-tum)
The extension of midbrain covering at the level of the pons.

pop culture USA
Refers to whatever is "hot"—such as fashion, movies, music, or lingo in North American marketing; refers to what is highly influential as *au courant* (in the "current") of culture.

pop semantics
Pertains to "spin" or whatever meaning the sender attaches to it.

pornography
Literally, "to write about prostitutes." Depicting erotic, sexual behavior, pictures, or text intended to cause sexual excitement.

pornography (hardcore)
Pornography rated XXX for violence, anal sex, bondage or sadomasochism. More explicit, varied, and perverted forms of pornography.

postmortem
Literally "after death."

postpartum
Literally, "after birth."

predator parenting
Refers to antisocial or toxic parenting.

prefrontal (cortex) lobes
Cortical regions in the frontal lobes thought to be involved in planning complex cognitive behavior, expression of personality, and appropriate social behavior.

prescient (prez-ee-unt)
Forward thinking.

proclivities (prok-liv-ugh-tees)
Inclination toward something objectionable

profiling
Pertains to gathering information at a crime scene in order to construct personality and other personal proclivities (habits and behavior) of an UNSUB.

profundity
Refers to gravity or depth of a condition.

projective test
Refers to psychometrics (testing) aimed at disclosing "deeper" dynamics of unconscious conflict.

protocol
A detailed plan of a scientific procedure

pseudo-intellectual
Literally, "false" intellectual. A person who pretends to be intellectual by using scholarly words.

pseudo-sapien
Literally, "false" sapient. Refers to a brain damaged sexual predator, who is not psychotic, but acts irrationally and criminally by preying upon others.

psyche (Seye-kee)
Greek word meaning "soul".

psychiatric social worker
Refers to a professionally trained person who is often part of a psychiatric treatmet team who specializes in family dynamics and pathological influences that threaten to disrupt normal interactions.

psycho-behavioral profile
Older term for criminal profiling denoting the importance of psychological principles and behavioral analysis in construction of the profiles.

psychobabble
Refers to using terms and concepts related to psychology in everyday conversation.

psychological perspectives
Psychological "schools" of thought—such as behaviorism or cognitive neuroscience—used in analyzing personality, behavior, or mind.

psychopathic personality (psychopath)
Severe emotional and behavioral state characterized by clear perception of reality except for social and moral obligations, which are overridden by the pursuit of immediate personal gratification in criminal acts, drug addiction, or sexual perversion.

psychopathology (sigh-ko-path-ology)
Refers to dysfunctional or deviant influences upon behavior such as disordered family dynamics, drug dependency, and aberrant thinking and how they influence the observation and documentation of abnormal behavior.

psychopathy
Pertains to psychopathic personality, psychopathic features, or in the extreme, sexual psychopathy.

psychosocial history
A clinical document prepared usually by a social worker detailing the family dynamics of a client seeking therapy.

psychotic
Pertains to insanity

psychotropic
Psychoactive medication that influences mood and/or behavior.

purposive behaviorism
Edward Tolman's "school" of behaviorism related to goal-directed behavior.

pyromania
An irresistible impulse to start fires.

Q

QM (quantum mechanics)
Quantum mechanics pertains to the structure, motion, and interaction of particles (atoms and molecules) where the discrete nature of the physical world is unimportant in contrast to classical physics.

R

RAS (reticular activation system)
A midbrain collection of medial nuclei important in regulation of sleep, motor activity, and diffuse integrative functions.

radical behaviorism
Refers to Skinnerian principles of operant conditioning without regard to mentalistic concepts.

"Rambo" killers
Adolescent kids who kill peers and adults in home and schoolplace violence.

rapacious (rugh-PAY-shus) {or **rapacity**} (rugh-PIS-ugh-tee)
Preying upon a victim by a perpetrator with intent to do physical bodily harm (such as rape or murder in sexual psychopathy) or to inflict psychological harm (as observed in brainwashing).

rape kit
Pertains to accessories brought to the crime scene by the perpetrator (such as duct tape and/or rope) to incapacitate the victim.

rationalism
The use of reason over emotion in perceiving and handling conflict.

rationalization
Freudian defense against anxiety by making "convincing" reasons to explain behavior.

reptilian brain (or reptilian brain theory)
Refers to the brain stem or R-complex (reptilian complex) as one of three overlapping brains purposed by neurologist Paul MacLean, former Chief of brain evolution and behavior at the National Institute of Health. The R-complex brain is closely related to physical survival, ritualistic behavior, and dominance.

resolution phase
In Masters and Johnson's human sexual response, the return to pre-arousal psychophysiological state.

rootedness
Pertains to feeling emotionally grounded and safe.

ruse
To deceive.

S

S→R psychology
In behaviorism, the reliance on cause and effect as determining behavior, presented as stimulus→response.

SSRIs (selective serotonin reuptake inhibitors)
Refers to the chemical action of blocking reuptake (liberating) serotonin in brain chemistry.

sadist (SAY-dist)
Pertains to the sexual perversion of feeling stimulation by inflicting pain or causing another to suffer.

sadomasochism (SAY-doe-mass-ugh-kiz-um)
Being sexually stimulated by both giving and receiving pain.

schizophrenia (skitz-ugh-free-nee-ugh)
Refers to a serious mental disorder characterized by a thought disorder and disintegration of personality.

schizotypal personality disorder (skezz-ugh-tie-pull)
In the DSM, a pervasive personality disorder characterized by acute discomfort with, and a reduced capacity for, close relationships, as well as by cognitive or perceptual distortions and eccentricities of behavior.

second messenger peptides (or **second messengers**)
Type of neurotransmitter that prolongs and modulates mood and emotion in contrast to fast acting ion-channeled linked receptors.

secondary follower role
Pertains to a person working in tandem as an accomplice with a serial killer

serial
Sequential, or one act following another act with a time lapse in between.

serial killer
Refers (usually) to a male killer in his twenties to mid-thirties characterized by sexual psychopathy, a violent subcategory comprising the larger classification of antisocial personality disorder and psychopathic personality. He kills at least three victims in sequence with a "cooling off" period—time spent away from killing.

serotonin (5-HT) (SARA-toe-none)
Powerful inhibitory neurotransmitter producing a calm, cool, and collected mood.

sex addict
Pertains to a person who is addicted to sexual stimulation and the accompanying brain chemistry lying behind the feeling.

sexual dysfunction NOS
Pertains to sexual dysfunctions that do not meet the criteria for any specific sexual dysfunction such as diminished erotic feelings or whether or not a sexual dysfunction is due to a general medical condition or substance induced.

sexual psychopathy (sighk-op-ugh-thee) or **sexual psychopath**
Extreme mental disorder marked by irrationality, perverted sexuality, egocentrism, and antisocial behavior. Viewed as the personality type of serial killers.

sexual sadism
Erotic desire caused by inflicted pain upon another.

shaken baby syndrome
Neurological damage to delicate brain tissue due to vigorously shaking the body of an infant.

signature
Refers to the emotional reason evidenced at the crime scene as the "calling card" that drives serial crime. It's what "jazzes" him everytime he commits the crime.

skepticism
A philosophical appeal of doubt and to gather more information before a conclusion is drawn. Educated doubt.

social modeling
Pertains to observational learning—watching and copying the behavior and mannerisms of others.

sodomized (sodomy)
Pertains to various forms of sexual intercourse considered unnatural or abnormal, especially anal intercourse or bestiality.

spree killer
Pertains (usually) to a male killer who kills in two or more locations with no "cooling off" period between kills.

staging
Following a crime, the placement of the body in a certain position by the perpetrator or family members in anticipation of the body being discovered.

sublimation
Freudian term relating to the redirection of libido away from pure sexuality into alternative social pursuits and achievements such as art and science.

substantia nigra (sub-stan-sugh-Neye-grugh)
Literally "black substance", part the basal ganglia and a rich source of dopamine.

subterfuge
Dishonesty.

successive approximations
The "small steps," or increments of behavior, required to shape (or perfect) behavior, such as the "small steps" of behavior are developed in hitting a baseball.

sui generis
Literally "of its own kind." Constituting a unique class alone.

surrogate
A substitute.

T

tableaux mortido
Literally "death pictures".

tactile stimulation
Refers to touch.

taxonomy
General principles observed in systematic classification (such as the Periodic Tables).

testosterone (Tess-tos-tugh-rone)
Powerful anabolic steroid; hormone of aggression and libido.

thalamus
Brain structure responsible for integration of sensory information from lower centers to higher centers of the brain.

toxic parenting
Pertains to antisocial parenting.

trephination (Tref-ugh-nay-shun)
Ancient medical practice of perforating the skull (such as drilling holes).

U

UNSUB
Refers to an unidentified subject in FBI lingo.

V

vasopressin (Vazo-pres-n)
Hormone secreted by the posterior pituitary gland that increases blood pressure, urine flow, and social bonding in males.

vignette (vin-yet)
Pertains to a short, descriptive literary sketch

voyeurism (voy-your-iz-um)
Literally "one who sees." Obtaining sexual gratification from viewing nudity or sexual acts; one who habitually seeks sexual gratification from visual means.

W

wolffian ducts (wolf-un ducks)
Pertains to tiny embryonic ducts responsible for male sexual differentiation under the influence of testosterone.

Z

zeitgeist (zeye-geye-st)
Literally "spirit of the times." The moral and intellectual climate in a given time in history as it impacts society and popular culture.

References

Adams, R. D., and Victor, M. *Principles of Neurology,* 5th ed. New York: McGraw-Hill, 1993.

American Psychiatric Association Diagnostic and Statistical Manual of Mental Disorders (4th Ed). DSM-IV-TR (2002). Washington, DC: American Psychiatric Association Press, 2002.

Barlow, David & Durand, V. Mark. *Abnormal Psychology,* 2nd ed. Belmont, California: Wadsworth, 2001.

Beatty, Jackson. *Principles of Behavioral Neuroscience.* Dubuque, Iowa: Brown & Benchmark, 1995.

Bugliosi, Vincent. *Outrage.* New York: Island Books, 1995.

Burgess, A. & Douglas, J. & Ressler, R., Eds. *Sexual Homicide: Patterns and Motives,* New York: Lexington Books, 1988.

Burgess, A. & Douglas, J. & Ressler, R. Eds. *Crime Classification Manuel,* San Francisco: Jossey-Bass Publishers, 1997.

Charles Manson: Journey into Evil. A & E Biography Videocassette. Arts & Entertainment. (1995).

Cohen, Sidney. *The Chemical Brain.* Irvine, California: CareInstitute, 1988.

Cooper, Jack R., Bloom, Floyd E., & Roth, Robert H. *The Biochemical Basis of Neuropharmacology,* 6th Ed. Oxford: Oxford University Press, 1991.

Douglas, John E., Olshaker, M. (1996). *Mind Hunter,* New York: Pocket Books.

Douglas, John E., Olshaker, Mark. *Obsession.* New York: Scribner, 1998.

Douglas, John E., Olshaker, M. *The Anatomy of Motive,* New York: Scribner, 1999.

Douglas, Ressler, Burgess, and Hartman. "Criminal Profiling from Crime Scene Analysis." *Behavioral Science and the Law,* 1986, 4-401–406.

Erikson, E. H. *Identity: Youth in Crisis.* New York: W. W. Norton, 1968.

Erikson, E. H. *The Life Cycle Completed: A Review.* New York: W. W. Norton, 1982.

Everitt, David. *Human Monsters.* Chicago: Contemporary Books, 1993.

Emmons, Nuel. *Manson: In His Own Words,* New York: Grove Press, 1986.

Films for the Humanities and Sciences. *Mind of a Murderer 2. Damaged: When Trauma Leads to Violence.* Princeton, N.J., 2002.

Films for the Humanities & Sciences. *Mind of Murderer 2. Men: The Killer Sex.* Princeton, N. J., 2002.

Films for the Humanities & Sciences. *Psychopaths: Natural Born Killers?* Princeton, N.J., 2002.

Films for the Humanities & Sciences. *The Mind of a Serial Killer.* Princeton, N.J., 1992.

Freeman, Lucy. *Before I Kill More,* New York: Crown Publishers, 1955.

Freud, Sigmund. *An Outline of Psychoanalysis.* In Standard Edition of the Complete Works of Sigmund Freud (Vol. 23). London: Hogarth Press, 1938.

Freud, Sigmund. *Civilization and its discontents.* College Edition. New York: W.W. Norton, 1961.

Gay, Peter. *Freud: A Life for Our Time.* New York: W. W. Norton, 1990.

Greenberg, Jerrold S., Bruess, Clint E., Mullen, Kathleen D. Dubuque, Iowa: Brown & Benchmark, 1992.

Haas, Kurt & Haas, Adelaide. *Understanding Sexuality* (3rd Ed.). St. Louis: Mosby, 1993.

Hare, Robert D. *Without Conscience.* New York: Guilford Press, 1999.

Harlow, H. F., Zimmerman, R. R. "Affection Responses in the Infant Monkey." *Science,* 1959. 130, 421–432.

Hock, Roger, R. *Forty Studies That Changed Psychology* (3rd ed.). New Jersey: Prentice Hall, 1999.

Holmes, Ronald M., and Holmes, Stephen T. *Profiling Violent Crimes: An Investigative Tool,* California: Sage Publications, 1999.

Horgan, John. *Rational Mysticism.* New York: Houghton Mifflin, 2003.

Hunt, Morton M. *The Story of Psychology*. New York: Doubleday, 1993.

Isenberg, Sheila. *Women Who Love Men Who Kill*. New York: Simon & Schuster, 1991.

Jack the Ripper: Phantom of Death. A & E Biography Videocassette. Arts & Entertainment, 1995.

Jacobs, Don. *Inside the Clinical Picture* (3rd ed.). Dubuque, Iowa: Kendall/Hunt Publishing, 2002.

Jacobs, Don. *Personality: Compositions of Mind*. Boston: McGraw-Hill, 2002.

Jacobs, Don. *Psychology: Brain, Behavior, and Popular Culture* (4th ed.). Dubuque, Iowa: Kendall/Hunt Publications, 2002.

Jacobs, Don. *Psychology of Adjustment* (3rd ed.). Dubuque, Iowa: Kendall/Hunt Publishers, 2002.

James, William. *The Varieties of Religious Experience*. New York: Collier, 1961.

Kennedy, Dolores. *Bill Heirens: His Day in Court,* Chicago: Bonus Books, 1991.

Keppel, Robert, D. *Signature Killers*. New York: Pocket Books, 1997.

Masters, W. H., Johnson, V. E. & Kolodny, R.C. *Human Sexuality*. Boston: Little, Brown, 1982.

Merriam-Webster, *Webster's Medical Desk Dictionary*. Massachusetts: Merriam-Webster, (1986).

Millenson, J. R. & Leslie, Julian C. *Principles of Behavioral Analysis* (2nd ed.). New York: McMillan, 1979.

Neitzel, M. *Crime and Its Modification: A Social Learning Perspective*. Elmsford, New York: Pergamon, 1979.

Norris, Joel. *Serial Killers,* New York: Anchor Books, 1988.

Ornstein, Robert. *The Roots of Self*. San Francisco: HarperCollins, 1995.

Peck, M. Scott. *The Road Less Traveled*. New York: Simon & Schuster, 1978.

Purves, Dale, et. al. Eds. *Neuroscience* (2nd ed.). Sunderland, Massachusetts: Sinauer Associates, 2001.

Ressler, Robert K., Shachtman, Tom. *Whoever Fights Monsters*. New York: St. Martin's, 1992.

Restak, Richard M. *Receptors*. New York: Bantam Books, 1995.

Russell, Bertrand. *A History of Western Philosophy*. New York: Simon & Schuster, 1945.

Siegel, Larry J. *Criminology* (8th ed.). Belmont, California: Wadsworth, 2003.

Skinner, B. F. *Science and Human Behavior*. New York: Macmillan, 1953.

Skinner, B.F. *Beyond Freedom and Dignity*. New York: Bantam Books, 1971.

Sundberg, Norman D. & Winebarger, Allen A. & Taplin, Julian R. *Clinical Psychology: Evolving Theory, Practice, and Research*. New Jersey: Prentice Hall, 2002.

The Wrong Man? PrimeTime Video, ABC Television, aired August 7, 1996.

Turvey, Brent. *Criminal Profiling: An Introduction to Behavioral Evidence Analysis,* London: Academic Press, 1999.

Watson, J. B. (1919). *Psychology from the Standpoint of a Behaviorist*. Philadelphia: Lippincott.

Watson, J. B. (1930). *Behaviorism*. New York: W. W. Norton.

Wormser, Rene A. (1962). *The Story of Law*. New York: Simon & Schuser.

Wrightsman, Nietzel, & Fortune (1997). *Psychology and the Law* (4th ed.). NY: Brooks/Cole Publishers.

Serial Homicide Websites

www.apt213.com

www.aristotle.net

www.courttv.com

www.crimelibrary.com

http://www.galenpress.com/demon_doctors

http://www.crimelibrary.com/serial_killers/predators/heirens/heirens_1.html

INTERPOL, *http://www.interpol.int*

www.paloaltodailynews.com

http://www.4degreez.com/misc/personality_disorder_test.mv

http://mentalhelp.net/poc/center_index

www.serialhomicide.com

www.serialkillers

Related Websites

http://www.corbis.com (Type in Name of Serial Killer)
Click here: Serial Murder

Click here: The Neuropathology of (Violent) Aggression

Click here: Types of Disorders: Sexual Disorders, including sexual dysfunctions, paraphilias, and gender identity disorders

Click here: Special: Violence as a Biomedical Problem

http://www.crimelibrary.com/

http://www.zodiackiller.com

http://www.courttv.com

http://www.carpenoctem.tv

http://serialkillers.coolbegin.com

runram50@yahoo.com

http://www.fortunecity.com/roswell/streiber/273/index.html

http://www.criminalprofiling.ch

http://flash.lakeheadu.ca/~pals/forensics

http://faculty.ncwc.edu/toconnor/401/401lect11.htm

http://www.crimelibrary.com/serial_killers/predators/index.html

Suggested Reading List

Book	Author(s)
A to Z Serial Killers	Harold Schechter and David Everitt
The Cases That Haunt Us	John Douglas and Mark Olshaker
Mindhunter	John Douglas and Mark Olshaker
Signature Killers	Robert D. Keppel and William J Birnes
I Have Lived in the Monster	Robert K. Ressler and Tom Shachtman
Jeffrey Dahmer	Joel Norris
The Evil That Men Do	Stephen G. Michaud with Roy Hazelwood
Dark Dreams	Roy Hazelwood and Stephen G. Michaud

Serial Killers—The Insatiable Passion	Joel Norris
Inside the Criminal Mind	Stanton E. Samenow
Step Into My Parlor—Serial Killer Jeffrey Dahmer	Ed Baumann
Serial Killers	David Lester
Alone with the Devil	Ronald Markman, M.D. and Dominick Bosco
Casebook of a Crime Psychiatrist	James A. Brussel, M.D.
Why They Kill	Richard Rhodes
Tears of Rage	John Walsh
Texas Crime Chronicles	Editors of Texas Monthly
William Heirens: His Day in Court	Dolores Kennedy
I Know You Really Love Me— *A Psychiatrist's of Obsessive Love*	Doreen Orion, M.D.
Helter Skelter: The Manson Murders	Vincent Bugliosi
Before I Kill More	Lucy Freeman
Basic Instincts—What Makes Killers Kill	Jonathan H. Pincus M.D.
And Deliver Us From Evil	Mike Cochran
Cracking Cases	Dr. Henry C. Lee and Thomas W. O'Neal
Evil—Inside Human Violence & Cruelty	Roy F. Baumeister, Ph.D.
Will You Die For Me?	Charles "Tex" Watson
Psychology of Crime	S. Giora Shoham and Mark Seis
Dead Man Walking	Sister Helen Prejean
Portrait of a Killer: Jack the Ripper	Patricia Cornwell
The Boy Next Door	Gretchen Brinck
A Father's Story	Lionel Dahmer
In Cold Blood	Truman Capote
The Killers Among Us	Colin Wilson and Damon Wilson
Defending the Devil—My Story as *Ted Bundy's Lawyer*	Polly Nelson
The Phantom Prince—My Life with Ted Bundy	Elizabeth Kendall
A Love to Die For	Patricia Springer
Blood Rush	Patricia Springer
Kids Who Kill	Charles Patrick Ewing
Guilt By Reason of Insanity	Dorothy O. Lewis, M.D.
Profiles in Murder	Russell Vorpagel
Famous Crimes Revisited	Dr. Henry C. Lee and Dr. Jerry Labriola